MEDIEVAL PLANTS
AND THEIR USES

MEDIEVAL PLANTS

AND THEIR USES

MICHAEL BROWN

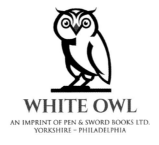

WHITE OWL

AN IMPRINT OF PEN & SWORD BOOKS LTD.
YORKSHIRE – PHILADELPHIA

First published in Great Britain in 2023 by
White Owl
An imprint of
Pen & Sword Books Ltd
Yorkshire - Philadelphia

ISBN 978 1 52679 458 1

Typeset in 11/14 pts Cormorant Infant
by SJmagic DESIGN SERVICES, India.

Printed and bound in India by Replika Press Pvt. Ltd.

Pen & Sword Books Ltd incorporates the imprints of Pen & Sword Books Archaeology, Atlas, Aviation, Battleground, Discovery, Family History, History, Maritime, Military, Naval, Politics, Railways, Select, Transport, True Crime, Fiction, Frontline Books, Leo Cooper, Praetorian Press, Seaforth Publishing, Wharncliffe and White Owl.

For a complete list of Pen & Sword titles please contact

PEN & SWORD BOOKS LIMITED
47 Church Street, Barnsley, South Yorkshire, S70 2AS, England
E-mail: enquiries@pen-and-sword.co.uk
Website: www.pen-and-sword.co.uk

or

PEN AND SWORD BOOKS
1950 Lawrence Rd, Havertown, PA 19083, USA
E-mail: Uspen-and-sword@casematepublishers.com
Website: www.penandswordbooks.com

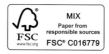

Contents

Foreword

I have always been interested in how plants have been chosen for so many different uses throughout history. When I created a medieval garden at the Prebendal Manor in Nassington, Northamptonshire, I chose plants as much for their use as their beauty. Consulting early books, I followed instructions to learn how people had used plants in the past. Not all my experiments were successful, but I became better at some with practice. Much of the written plant-lore of Europe dates to classical Greece and Rome. Many editions of the translated texts are difficult to come by. I have tried to combine medieval and contemporary texts to bring the main uses of plants together. The folklore and myths are included as the understanding of the relationship of the plant to the people of the time cannot be fully understood unless we have as much information as possible. This book brings together some of my research, in what I hope is an easy to understand and enjoyable manner. This is only an introduction, the start of an adventure that can lead you to many new places.

Disclaimer

Never try to diagnose and treat your own medical condition or that of others. Just because a herb is natural and was used in the past, it does not mean that it is considered safe to use today. Many of the plants in the book can cause injury or death. Be aware that the sap of some plants, such as *Ruta* and *Euphorbia* can cause skin rashes and blistering.

All of the following recipes are for historical interest only. The author and publisher accept no liability for any injury caused by any use of the plants and methods included in this book.

CHAPTER 1

Introduction

Plants were an essential part of medieval life. When examining the plants that were used during the medieval period, it soon becomes apparent that there were very few plants that did not have any use at all, although today many of them would be considered as weeds.

Food, medicines, dyes and cosmetics are uses that first come to mind. Less obvious is housing, with many houses being mostly constructed using wood and thatch.

In the home, lots of wood was burned to provide warmth and to cook food. More wood was then required to make furniture and a huge variety of containers, drinking vessels, plates and spoons. Outside, the gardener's spade was wood with only a metal sheath on the end to make digging easier; the rake and dibber were also made of wood. Wood was used by armies to construct siege machines, shields, bows, arrows and weapon handles along with the carts that were needed to transport all the equipment. Boats and ships were used for local and distant travel. Singing and dancing were enjoyed by many, and most of the musical instruments were made of wood. The practical uses of plants are seemingly endless.

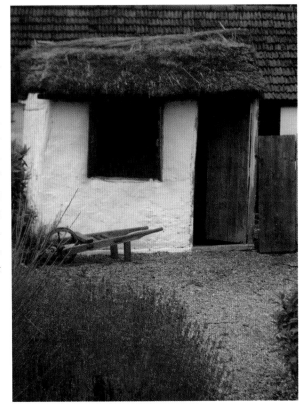

A replica medieval thatched hut built using wooden beams, wattle and daub.

Most people today when asked about medieval plant use will think of herbs. What *is* a herb? During the medieval period and later, the word herb, or *wort*, simply meant a plant. The usual definition of a herb is that it is any plant that is of use to humankind, whether it is eaten, used medicinally, or as a cosmetic; we could include other uses. Many herbs traditionally have several uses, and lots of them have decorative or aromatic qualities that make them good garden plants for a modern garden.

The scientists of ancient Greece recorded many of the plants that they used, noting their properties in herbals that describe the plant and give various uses. These books were copied by the Romans, who later wrote about their own discoveries. Herbals survived the fall of the Roman Empire to re-emerge into common use through the monastic system and medical schools and plant and medicinal knowledge benefited from the Arabic writers translating ancient texts. Once herbals were being used again, medieval writers often simply repeated the ancient authors. Some writers did include their own observations, and in some cases, criticised and contradicted the earlier writers, who had often catalogued the common knowledge and use of plants, rather than offering their own practical experience. The magical association of plants would survive the Renaissance, and in the case of lunar planting, they would periodically return, like the moon, even into the twenty-first century.

The Pleasure Gardens of the wealthy grew many plants for colour, scent, and texture for enjoyment only. The plants in the pleasure garden were not for use, they were allowed to flourish and bloom and fade away without being cut for either the kitchen or for medicnes; although plants were grown for use in another garden. Elsewhere, most people were growing the same plants as useful herbs, for practical purposes, rather than just for pleasure. Plants were used medicinally to make you well, or to ease pain. Many cosmetics were plant based, with beauty treatments to remove freckles, rough skin and to lighten the skin colour. Equally popular were the recipes to prevent hair loss and for colouring it. Many plants had a more practical benefit. Linen cloth was made from plant fibres, coloured using plant dyes and could be cleaned using soapwort.

CHAPTER 2

Medieval Vegetables

Many of the culinary plants and flavourings have survived in use into the present time, although most of them have been improved using selective breeding to produce greater yields. Some plants are still grown decoratively in gardens but are no longer in general use, as fashions, tastes and medical knowledge have changed over the centuries.

For most people in the past, plants were grown for food. The diet for the majority of the medieval population was based on plants that they grew themselves. During periods of famine, people would be forced to forage for food, but there were quite a few hungry gaps during most years, even without any fasts imposed by the church. Monks were mostly vegetarian, especially in the earlier periods, but are recorded as eating much more fish and meat towards the end of the medieval period until the Reformation. Dwellings in both the country and the towns usually had a good-sized garden that would enable you to keep chickens and maybe a pig, with more space to grow plants for food, cosmetics, and medicine.

It used to be thought that the medieval upper-classes did not eat vegetables. This was mostly due to the place meat was given as a status symbol and because the expense accounts for many different meats for festive occasions rarely mention vegetables. Meat eating was very much dependent on your status in life and some meats such as venison and boar were esteemed for their cultural value as much as their taste. Vegetables were considered the main food source for the lower classes, but they were grown by secular and religious households. For vegetables that were being grown in England and for practical gardening advice we have John Gardener, who wrote in English rather than Latin. He suggested that we should grow a variety of culinary plants, as well as some of the medicinal ones, in his poem, now known as, *The Feate of Gardenynge*. The surviving manuscript dates to about 1440 but may have been written earlier. Gardener recommends successive sowing to ensure a good supply of each plant throughout the year. He noted that the cabbage family, *Wortys*, were eaten 'by both master and knave'. The wealthy were eating vegetables at high status banquets, most likely supplied from the household's own garden. For all classes, vegetables would be in shorter supply during the winter months. The recipes that have survived are those of the higher end of the social scale, giving us some idea of the vegetables, fruit and grains that were being eaten by the wealthy. The recipes usually list the ingredients and methods to be used, but rarely include quantities as the overall flavour and the seasoning was to be adjusted to suit your own personal taste.

Broad Beans, *Vicia faba*, and Peas, *Pisum sativum*, have been in cultivation for millennia. Beans were grown in Egypt since 1800 BCE and have been in Europe for about two thousand years. Peas have been cultivated for longer than beans, but do not appear to have been grown in England until the Norman conquest. Beans and peas were reliable sources of protein for the lower classes. They are easy to grow and store with the advantage that a few nibbles by various pests will not make them inedible, and they can be kept for long periods of time without deteriorating. Both were added to pottage, a vegetable based stew that was the main part of the daily diet for many people. It is a vegetable broth made with dried beans or peas with whatever vegetables and flavourings are in season. Meat or fish could be added if you have them. Pottage as a daily staple may sound tedious, but the flavour would change throughout the year as different plants became available. Beans and peas were part of the crop rotation of the time; the roots of both plants have root nodules that fix free-atmospheric nitrogen to their roots, which added nitrogen to the soil as the roots decomposed. The scientific process may not have been understood by earlier people, but the practical advantages had certainly been observed and were used.

Beans and peas could be ground to make a flour which was sometimes added to bread flour when grains were in short supply. Beans and peas stems were harvested when the pods had dried. They would be stored in barns and later threshed to remove the seeds. The left-over dried stems were not wasted, being used for animal fodder

A RECIPE TO COOK BEANS

Remove the beans from the pods. Without soaking them, put the beans into a pan on the fire until skins are wrinkled. Move the pan from the fire and carefully take the skins off the beans. Put the beans in cold water and heat until they burst. Remove the water and drain, add meat broth if it is a meat day, add oil and well-cooked onions that were then fried in butter. The puree can be fried or served as it is.

Beans have the unfortunate side effect of flatulence. One traditional way of countering this was to cook them with the evergreen herb Winter Savory.

Peas and beans were the staple diet of the religious orders, especially in the stricter, earlier period, leading to one monk's complaint that, 'Yesterday I had peas and pot herbs, today pot herbs and peas; tomorrow I shall eat peas with my pot herbs and the day after pot herbs with my peas.'

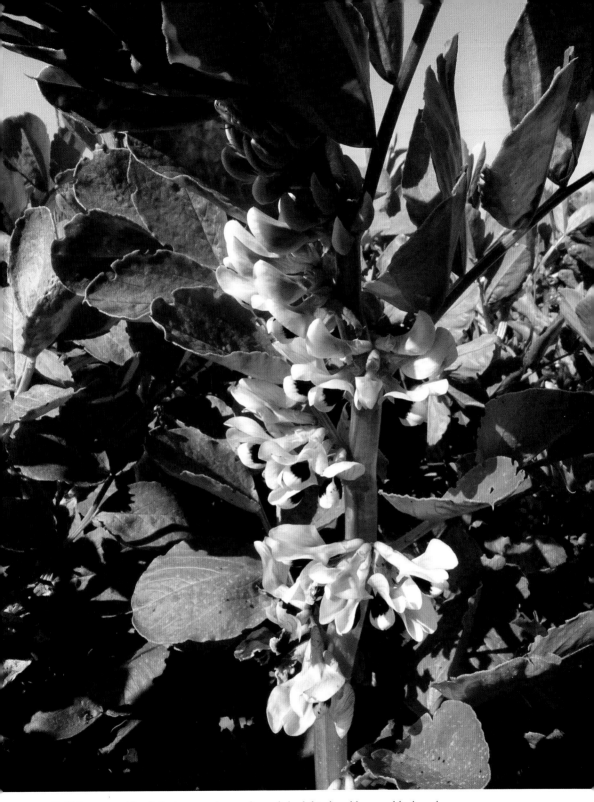

Field Beans would only be harvested once the pods had dried and become blackened.

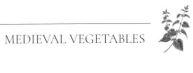

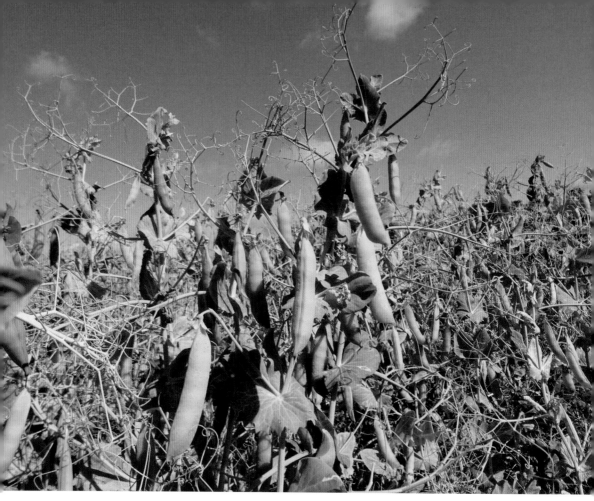
Peas were dried as an ingredient for pottage.

The following recipe shows that the peas were stored in their shells until ready for use.

DRIED PEA POTTAGE

Shell the peas, then without soaking soaking the dried peas, boil them in fresh water until they burst. Change the water and boil again. Then empty the water and simmer the peas without added water. Shake the pot but do not stir with a spoon, then adding a little hot water at a time, heat until thoroughly cooked. You can then add meat. On fish days, fish and onions are cooked in separate pots. Cook the onions for as long as the peas. Add the water from the onions to the peas, then fry the onions and mix them into the peas. Add salt as desired.

Leafy vegetables would add flavour and bulk to the pottage. Most of the leafy vegetables would be grown as cut-and-come-again crops, the mature leaves being removed from several plants. One whole plant would not be harvested by cutting

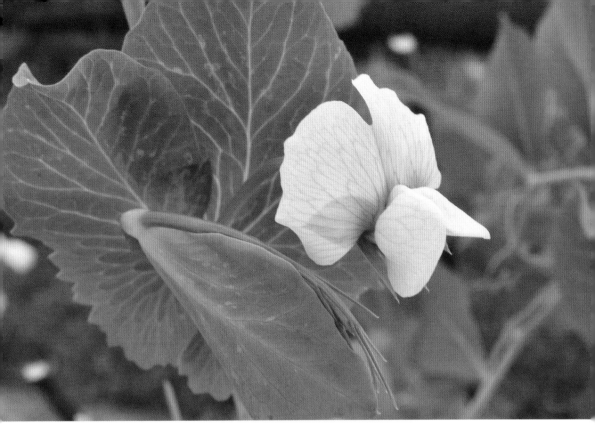

Pea flowers are attractive, so they could be grown as a decorative plant. They were often shown in the border of manuscript illustrations.

through the stem as we tend to today when cutting a cabbage for use. Cut-and-come-again is a labour-saving method of growing plants. You do not need to keep sowing seeds to replace harvested plants, nor do you have the work of watering seedlings as the summer progresses and the soil becomes drier. Medieval advice was not to remove leaves when the sun is hot, or the cuts would be burned, and the new leaves would not grow. The cabbage, *Brassica oleracea*, known as the *worty* or *colewort*, was one of the main leaf plants. Early cabbages tended to be more like a kale plant, not headed as modern cabbages are. Headed cabbage were known, but do not appear to have been reliable enough for general cultivation. Surplus early cabbage plants could be eaten as spring greens. With good planning, some form of cabbage would be available throughout the year. Grown as a cut-and come-plant these cabbages produced leaves for a long period. In modern Galicia in northern Spain, you can still see similar plants growing in rural gardens along with onions, garlic, and potatoes. All these vegetables are the staple ingredients of Caldo Gallego, the local stew which is the Galician version of pottage. There are many variations that include meat and beans. Caldo Gallego is made with whatever you have at hand. A medieval French recipe said that cabbages should be cooked over a hot fire from early morning for a long time, much more than any other leafy vegetable, preferably with a beef or mutton stock. Headed cabbage of red and white forms appear to have been available in England by the latter part of the fourteenth century. Red cabbage is mentioned in a fifteenth century book as an ingredient for an ointment to ease wounds. Two staples of modern cuisine, potatoes and tomatoes would not have been available in Britain during the medieval period.

AN ENGLISH RECIPE FOR CABBAGES

Cut the cabbage into quarters. Bring to the boil in a good broth (use a stock of your choice), then simmer. Add minced or finely chopped onions and the white part of leeks thinly sliced into rings. Season with salt, saffron and *powdour douce*, which is usually cinnamon and sugar ground finely with a pestle and mortar.

Other leaf vegetables were the several forms of beets. In some countries beets were grown mainly for their roots, and others for the leaves. Beets, *Beta vulgaris*, are very easy to grow and not so prone to bolting in dry weather as spinach. Good King Henry, *Chenopodium bonus-henricus*, often known today as Lincolnshire Spinach, is a perennial, so the leaves usually appear before vegetable seed that has been sown in spring; providing leaves for food when not much else is available. The leaves are slightly hairy and may not suit modern tastes. It is in the same family as Fat Hen, *Chenopodium vulgaris*, an annual plant whose leaves and seeds have been eaten since the Neolithic period. Purslane, *Portulaca, oleracea*, is not commonly grown now, but besides being eaten as a vegetable it had several medical uses. It was useful for agricultural workers during the summer as it was said that if you ate purslane, you would not be harmed by the heat of the sun. Lettuce, *Lactuca sativa*, has been grown and developed as a food since at least the Roman period. Lettuce does grow wild in Britain,

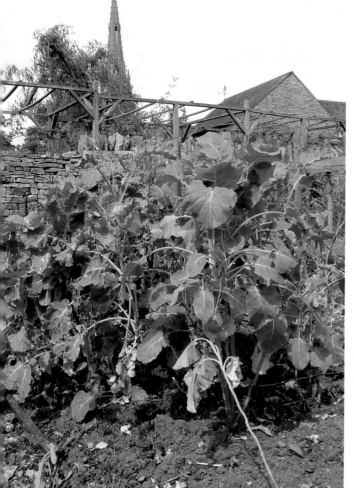

Wortys were grown for 'both master and knave'.

but the native lettuce has a very bitter taste and was usually used medicinally as a substitute for opium. Most of the medieval pictures of lettuce are from Italian produced copies of *Tancuinum Sanitatis*, a medical book produced for the general population, rather than medical professionals. The lettuce that are illustrated are shown as being similar to the Romaine type. Unfortunately, we can only guess at the appearance of the lettuce being grown in Britain during the medieval period. Herbals described lettuce as being cold and moist, so it could be used medicinally to cool the heat of a patient. Alexanders, *Smyrnium olusatrum*, were introduced by the Romans. They are still commonly seen growing wild at Roman sites such as Branodunum on the North Norfolk coast and along the local roadsides. The roots and leaves are edible, making it a useful plant to be grown in gardens as a vegetable.

Wild Celery, *Apium graveolens*, was grown for its leaves which could be used in pottage and sauces. It would not be until after the medieval period that the plant would be developed for its stems. Another herb with a celery-like flavour is lovage, *Levisticum officinale*, a tall perennial plant. Both the leaves and seeds could be added to pottage and other dishes. Other plants grown for their leaves include: sorrel, *Rumex acetosa*; orache, *Atriplex hortensis*; rocket, *Eruca sativa*; cress, *Lepidium sativum*; chicory, *Cichorium intybus*; and spinach, *Spinacia oleracea*. Many of these leaf plants have strong flavours and are not as tender as modern varieties, making them less palatable for many modern tastes.

Onions, *Allium cepa*, are not native to Britain but are now so ubiquitous that it is very hard to imagine the flavour of food without onions. The onion seems to have arrived in Britain with the Romans. Medieval accounts regularly record onions. Seed was bought, sown and the plants tended. Onions themselves were bought and sold if there was a surplus. The onion family are easy to grow and are a staple ingredient of pottage with all parts of the plant being used. Shallots, *Allium ascalonicum*, form

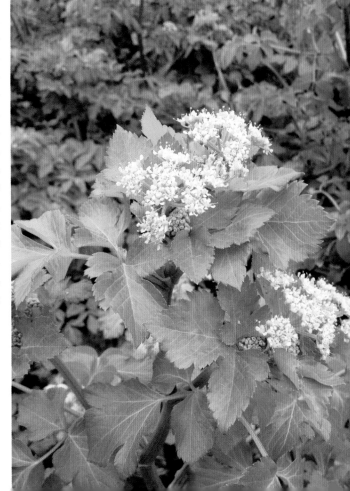

Alexanders continued to be grown as a vegetable after the Romans left Britain.

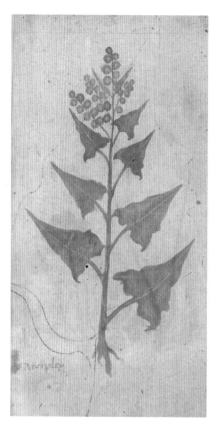

Orache is an annual plant that was grown as a leaf vegetable. (Wellcome Collection)

clumps of bulbs. They are usually grown from one bulb to produce a new clump, rather than from seed. Shallots tend to be a more reliable crop than onions. Garlic, *Allium sativum*, is also usually grown from a bulb to produce a clump. Garlic was popular in medieval England. It was used for food, medicine and to ward off evil. Leeks, *Allium porrum*, were a common plant, having been popular since the Anglo-Saxon period. The name *leac-garth* and *leac-tun* as a garden area occurs in many documents, which suggest that leeks were an important part of the diet at the time. During the medieval period, a distinction was made between green and white leeks. Green leeks were sown broadcast, scattering the seeds, rather than sowing in rows as is now common practice, and grown to maturity without any further work other than weeding. White leeks needed more labour. A trench could be dug with a mattock, the leeks transplanted, then the trench back-filled so that the lower stems would be blanched and become more tender than those of the green leeks. Only the wealthy with paid gardeners would have the time and facilities to grow the white leeks. Leeks are usually grown for use during the winter months, but if you are careful, it is possible to have leeks for much of the year. The Babington leek is a tall leek-like plant with a mild garlic flavour that can be found growing wild, but it is not certain whether it is native.

LEEK POTTAGE

Make almond milk by soaking two ounces of ground almonds in four cups of boiling water overnight and then straining the liquid through a sieve. Meanwhile, rinse white leeks in cold water and slice them thinly into rounds. Boil and drain to remove surplus water from the leeks. Mix the almond milk with breadcrumbs, then add the leeks and salt, with any other seasoning you wish. Simmer for five minutes or so. Add more water if it is too thick for you.

Another member of the onion family that is still grown for winter use is the Welsh Onion, *Allium fistulosum*, which is grown for the large hollow leaves which can be

MEDIEVAL PLANTS AND THEIR USES

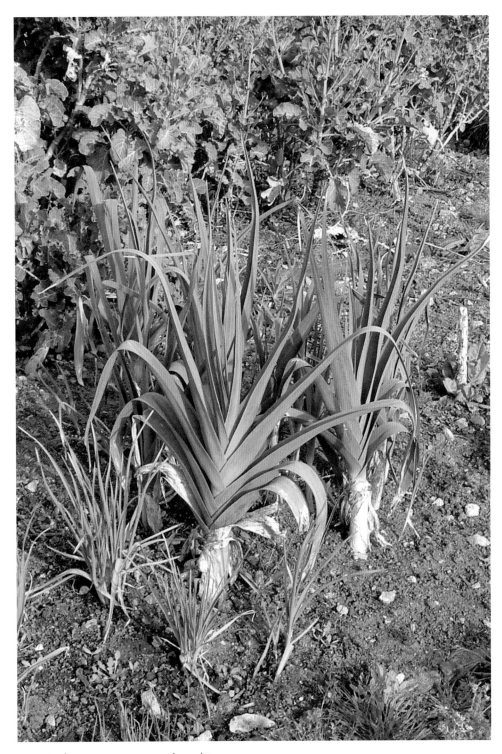

Green Leeks were easier to grow than white ones.

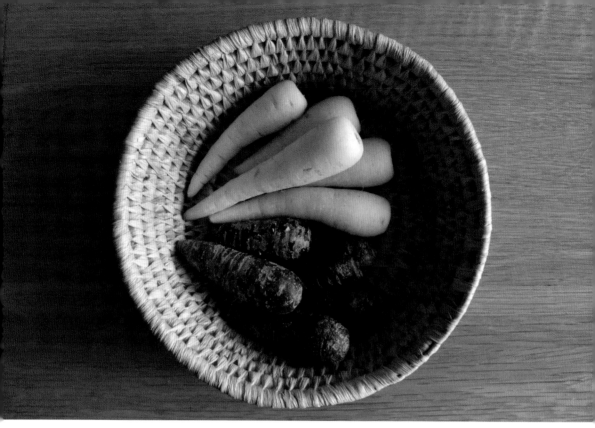

Carrots were of many colours other than orange.

treated as if they are large chives. Chives, *Allium schoenoprasum*, have a milder flavour than onions and can be left to grow with very little attention. The leaves begin to grow in the spring and can be cut off to flavour food. The purple flowers are edible, adding colour to a dish when they are sprinkled over food. Chives quickly self-seed all over the place and quickly produce new leaves as the old ones are cut off for use.

Garden grown root vegetables were fairly limited in number. Parsnips, *Pastinaca sativa*, had been grown since at least the Romans. They are probably the Neeps or Neps that occur in plant lists from the medieval period. Neps could possibly refer to turnips too, but we cannot be certain. Parsnip roots have a high sugar content and were served in many ways other than as a pottage plant. Parsnips may not have been widely used as they are fussy about the soil they are grown in to produce good crops.

Carrot, *Daucus carota*, is a plant native to Britain, with tapering white roots that are not generally very large. As a vegetable, carrots probably arrived as a benefit of the Crusades. The colours ranged from white, yellow, orange, red and purple. These carrots, with their sweet roots, soon became popular. They can be stored over winter in a frost-free environment and made a filling addition to the pottage. Recipes from cookery books show that they were favoured among the upper classes.

Skirrets, *Sium sisarum*, were grown for their roots and had been especially favoured by the Roman emperor, Tiberius, who ate them regularly. Skirrets were said to be warm and dry, but they were not to be eaten in excess or they would upset the stomach and cause fevers. They have a chequered history as a vegetable, going in and out of fashion at irregular intervals. The roots are quite small, so they are not the sort of food that would be grown by lower classes who may prefer to grow for quantity rather than quality, although in their favour, they are easy to grow by seed and division and require no special maintenance.

FRITTERS OF PARSNIPS, SKIRRETS AND APPLES

Parboil the parsnips, skirrets, and apples. Slice the apples and parsnips, but the skirrets are thin, so can be left whole. Make a batter of flour and eggs, with some saffron salt, ale and yeast. Allow the batter mix to rest for about an hour in a warm room. Dip the parsnips, skirrets and apples in the batter and fry them in oil or fat. You can serve with a sauce of almond milk.

Radish, *Raphanus sativus*, is mainly grown for its roots, but the leaves and seed pods are edible. There are many sorts of radish other than the quick to grow, round, red ones that are mostly sold in the shops. As with most medieval plants, it is impossible to know which sorts were being grown, but most radish have the hot, sharp flavour that was popular at the time. During periods of famine, roots such as Burdock could be gathered from the wild to supplement the diet.

One of the most important food flavourings, for the wealthy at least, was saffron, *Crocus sativus*. It was imported in huge amounts during the medieval period as many

Skirrets have small roots, so were most likely eaten by wealthier people.

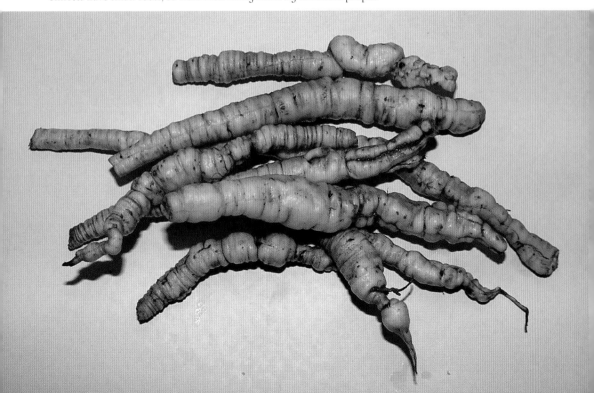

expense accounts of the time prove. The saffron spice is the stamens, of which there are only three per plant. It was eventually grown in England at places such as Saffron Walden, although this did little to reduce the reliance on imported saffron. It was very expensive and very much a plant for those with money to show off their status. Battle Abbey bought it by the sack full. It was not only used to flavour and colour food but produced a good dye and a paint. Medicinally, saffron was thought to be one of the better medicines to be used against the plague and was useful for treating tuberculosis.

Food flavours were enhanced using many of the herbs that we still use today, but they could be used to counter the perceived heat or coldness of foodstuffs; many had medicinal properties. Parsley, *Petroselinum crispum*, was a favourite herb and is frequently mentioned in recipes. It has a reputation of being difficult to germinate but once growing it can be productive for a long time if it is regularly cut for use. The leaves were used for their flavour and to colour food a bright green by pounding the leaves to a pulp. Eating parsley with food would make you well and assist digestion by drawing out the bad winds that were inside your body. It was also good for easing coughs.

Coriander, *Coriandrum sativum*, was as useful as parsley, with the bonus that the seed could be saved for use during the winter months when the plant was not growing in the garden. Today we grow the peony solely as a decorative plant, but the seeds were mentioned in the medieval poem, *Piers Plowman*, as a spice to flavour food. Oregano, *Origanum vulgare*, not only added flavour to food, it was a panacea for many ills! Drunk in a good white wine it would help your digestion after a large meal. It was suggested as an antidote for *Aconitum* poisoning. Oregano had the power to help the dumb to speak again, to improve your eyesight, stop earache, ease toothache, reduce fevers, increase urine, destroy worms in the stomach, cure the bites of venomous beasts and assist with myriad other problems. Oregano alone should have ensured that nobody was ever ill again, nor for long if they become ill! Sweet marjoram was recorded as being grown, but it was more difficult to grow in the English climate at the time. Mint is a very easy plant to grow. It thrives in most soils and spreads rapidly. One herbal stated the obvious, saying that if you planted mint, you would never be short of it, and that there were too many mints for any one man to name them all! Mint was popular as a flavouring, but could be used, as it still is today, to freshen the breath and to settle the stomach. Mint sauce made with vinegar was served to stimulate the appetite. Fennel, *Foeniculum vulgare*, and Dill, *Anethum graveolens*, can generally be treated as interchangeable in culinary recipes. Fennel comes up every year, so it is easier to grow than dill, which needs sowing every year. Both plants have a mild aniseed flavour that has been used with fish recipes since antiquity to counter the effects of oily fish on the stomach. Basil, *Ocimum basilicum*, is not a native plant of Britain, and was once again one more of the more useful things that the Romans did for us! Rocket, *Eruca sativa*, gives a bite to raw salads. It is an easy plant to grow for salads and as a flavouring for other foods, but as with many other food plants, it was credited with medicinal properties. White Mustard, *Sinapsis alba*, was commonly grown in medieval gardens. The pungent taste appealed to the palate of the time. It was grown in huge quantities, shown by the fact that in 1483, Norwich cathedral paid labourers to collect and thresh the mustard to remove the seeds. Norwich would become the main centre for mustard production in the early nineteenth century, but during the late medieval period Tewkesbury was famed for its mustard. The seeds were easy to store and keep for years. Mustard sauce requires the seeds to be crushed using a pestle and mortar, which is quite a laborious process. Mustard can also be made into balls, which in the days before cheap containers was an easy way to sell mustard or a way of having ready-prepared mustard ready for use.

MUSTARD BALLS

There is a lot of variation in mustard ball ingredients. Make to suit your own preferences.

When crushing by hand with a pestle and mortar, I first soak a quantity of mustard seeds in water, wine, or vinegar until they are soft. Crush the seeds to a smooth consistency, but some seeds can be left whole if you want a grittier texture. Dried fruits such as raisins or dates can be added and any other herbs or spices that you would like. Make the paste into balls and dry them in the sun or a warm room. The balls will keep for over a year. Break off pieces as needed, and mix with water, wine or vinegar to make a mustard paste or sauce.

Mustard Balls were an easy way of storing mustard for sauces.

Many of the herbs used for flavouring foods had medicinal qualities. For those who suffered when they ate cheese, whether cooked or not, cumin seed eaten with the cheese would prevent the problem. Chives could be served with fatty meats to prevent the queasy feeling that they can sometimes cause. Horseradish root, *Cochlearia armoracia*, which is popular today as a hot, piquant sauce with beef, does not appear to have reached Britain until the 1600s.

CHAPTER 3

Medieval Fruits and Nuts

Every large household that had enough land would possess an orchard to grow fruit and nuts. Local markets would provide an outlet for any surplus. Besides being of practical use, the orchard was also a place of beauty for relaxation and could be symbolic of the Garden of Eden, which had trees that were pleasant to view and bore fruit that was good for eating. Generally during the medieval period and for some time after, it was generally considered unhealthy and even potentially dangerous, to eat fruit fresh, except for strawberries and cherries, both being fruits that will be eaten by the blessed in heaven.

To sweeten cooked fruit the wealthy could add honey, but the cheapest sweetener for many people would be Sweet Cicely, *Myrrhis odorata*, which has an anise flavour. It is easy to grow and rapidly seeds around a garden.

Apples and pears were often made into cider and perry, with both drinks becoming more popular following the Norman Invasion. Apples had originally been domesticated in the Middle East. Later they were cultivated by the Romans, who very likely introduced their cultivated apples to Britain where only the wild crab apples grew naturally. The stock of cultivated apple varieties was quickly increased by grafting the cultivated apples onto the crab apple rootstocks. There were no dwarfing rootstocks, so fruit trees would have been taller than those seen now. With careful storage in cool, dry barns, late ripening apples can be kept over winter, providing fruit ready to hand for dessert dishes and sauces.

The wild pear is a small hard fruit that can sometimes be found growing in hedgerows. The fruit are very small, although the branches produce masses of white blooms in the spring. The disadvantage is that wild pear trees usually develop rather nasty thorns!

The domesticated pear, *Pyrus communis*, was known to the Romans although it is uncertain whether they introduced the pear to Britain. The best-known medieval pear is the Warden, which was thought to take its name from the Cistercian monastery at Old Warden, Bedfordshire. It is not a pear for eating fresh as the fruit is very hard, which means that it keeps well throughout the winter and into early spring. Wardens were cooked in several ways, sometimes using the same recipes as for the quince, which is also a very hard fruit.

MEDIEVAL PLANTS AND THEIR USES

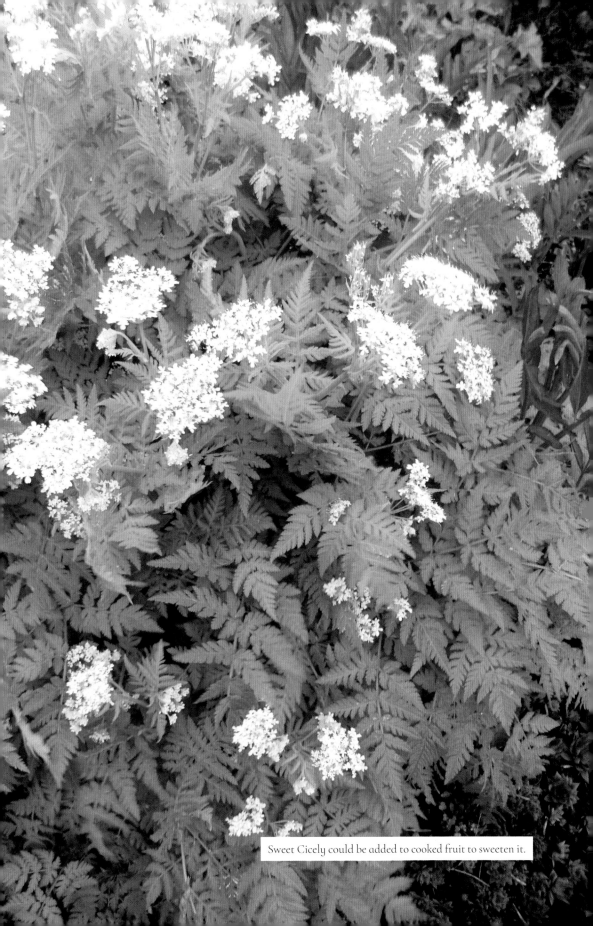

Sweet Cicely could be added to cooked fruit to sweeten it.

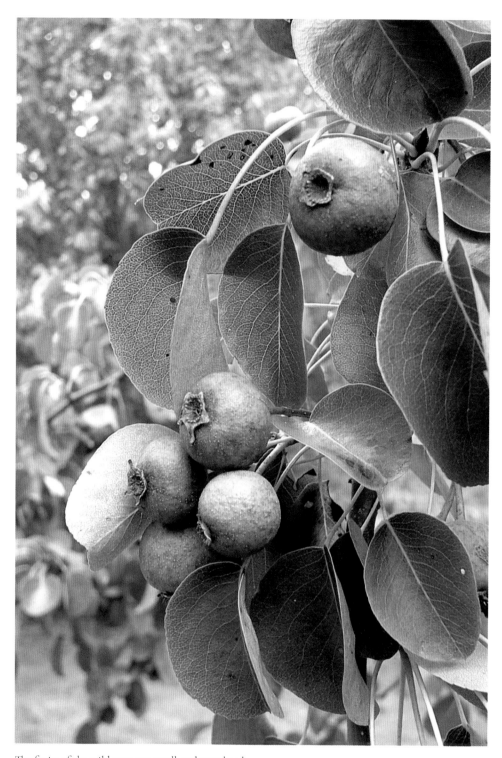

The fruits of the wild pear are small and very hard.

WARDONYS IN SYRUP

Take wardens, and put them in a pot, and boil them till they become tender; then take them out and pare them and cut them in two pieces. (It is uncertain whether the original recipe means into pieces, or in two pieces. I prefer the latter). Now take a good quantity of cinnamon powder and put it in red wine, and draw it through a strainer, then add sugar to it, and put it in an earthenware pot and bring it to the boil, then add the pears to the liquid, and boil them together. When they have boiled a while, take powdered ginger and put some in with a little vinegar and a little saffron. Check that it is poynaunt and sweet.

From the fifteenth century *Austin Manuscripts*

The quince grown during the medieval period, *Cydonia oblonga*, is no relation to the so-called Japanese Quince, *Chaenomeles speciosa*, which many people grow as a decorative shrub and has much smaller and rounder fruits. The true quince originates from ancient Persia and was grown throughout the Mediterranean. The tree is self-fertile but produces better fruit if cross-pollination can take place. Large white or pink flowers are followed by the fruit, which is similar to a very large pear, with a soft bloom over a skin that ripens to a deep golden yellow. The fruit develop such a heady fragrance that a single quince can scent a room. The fruit will ripen on the tree in a suitable climate but in Britain it rarely does, so they must be picked before the frosts begin. Quince was a popular fruit during the medieval period. You can cook them using a medieval recipe for pears, usually with wine and spices. The original marmalade was made with quinces. Because of the amount of sugar or honey, this would only be affordable for the wealthy.

QUINCE MARMALADE

Take the ripe quinces and quarter them. Do not remove the skin, core or pips. Boil them in a small quantity of water. Some recipes do not use any water at all. Push the pulp through a sieve. This is necessary to remove all the hard pieces. It is not an easy task. Do not be tempted to use food whizzer as it will not do the job properly! Weigh the pulp. Boil an equal weight of honey, removing any scum from the surface. Add the quince pulp then boil the mixture whilst continually stirring until the quantity is reduced by half and is moving from the sides of the pan. You may need a little more water to prevent burning. The pulp can be poured into shallow trays or decorative moulds to cool. It is best to let it dry for several days, until it becomes firm and chewy before putting in a sealed container.

I have made the recipe using the more modern method of substituting sugar for the honey. I kept one batch in a sealed container for over ten years. This recipe is

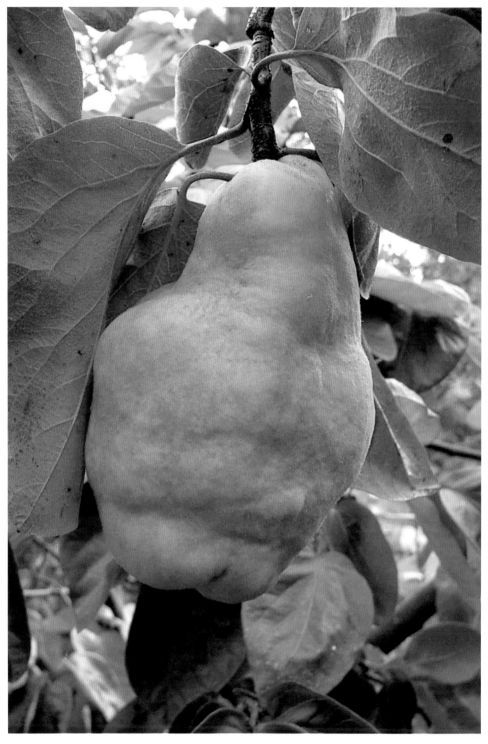

The Quince produces a large hard fruit.

MEDIEVAL PLANTS AND THEIR USES

essentially the same as for *Membrillo*, which is still sold in delicatessens at a very high price and is sometimes served with cheese plates at gourmet restaurants.

Medlars, *Mespilus germanica*, have been cultivated in Europe since at least the Roman period. The tree is self-fertile, so only one tree is required to produce fruit. The flowers are white or sometimes they have a flush of pale pink. The light brown fruit is like a small, flattened apple with an open end, which gave rise to its nickname, open-arse. The fruit does not usually ripen properly in Britain, remaining hard and quite acidic. In a cold climate the fruit needs to go through a process known as, *bletting*, to become edible. The unripe fruits can be picked in late October and stored in a cool, dry shed, although some people allow it to be exposed to a frost before harvesting. The fruit slowly becomes softer; the skin turns a dark brown and shrivels, whilst the inside becomes dark brown, and soft and squishy. After three weeks or so the fruit will be ready to eat. The inside is similar to a puree but be careful of the very large pips! The flavour is difficult to describe as it tastes like nothing else. As the fruit becomes rotten before it is ripe, the medlar was used figuratively in medieval literature as a symbol of prostitution or premature destitution. In the *Prologue* to *The Reeve's Tale*, Geoffrey Chaucer's character laments his old age, comparing himself to the medlar. 'Open-ers' refers to the fruit's nickname.

> This white top writeth myne olde yeris;
> Myn herte is mowled also as myne heris —
> But if I fare as dooth an open-ers.
> That ilke fruyt is ever lenger the wers,
> Til it be roten in mullok or in stree.
> We olde men, I drede, so fare we:
> Til we be roten, kan we nat be rype;

The mulberry tree, *Morus nigra*, tends to appear very ancient even from an early age. It will often lean or fall over and then re-grow from the base. The fruits are long and nearly cylindrical ripening to a dark black colour. If you try to pick or eat the ripe fresh fruit, your hands and mouth will be covered with the stains of the red juice, and you will be caught red-handed! The fruits were used to make wine. Thomas Becket's murderers are traditionally said to have left their cloaks and armour on a mulberry tree outside Canterbury cathedral. This mulberry is not the tree that provides the food for silkworms.

Cherries were one of the fruits the blessed would enjoy in heaven. One painting shows Saint Dorothy picking cherries in a heavenly garden. Back on earth, the cherry tree is usually the one shown in pictures where somebody is scrumping fruit. The temptation must have been very hard to resist for many children. The *Luttrel Psalter* shows a child up a cherry tree, his cheeks swollen with cherries as he is

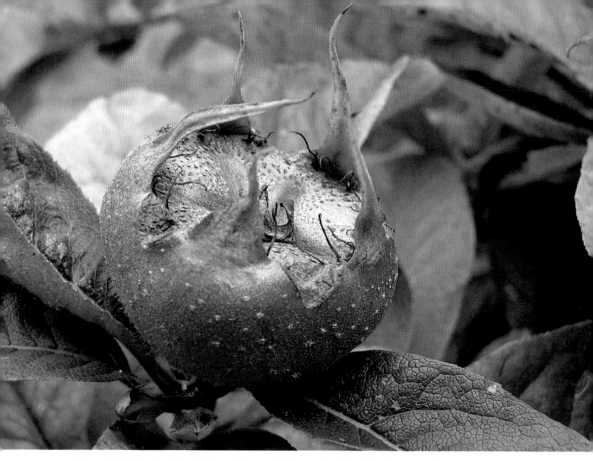

Above: In Britain, the fruit of the medlar usually has to be bletted before it can be eaten.

Below: Ripe Mulberries will leave you red-handed when you pick them.

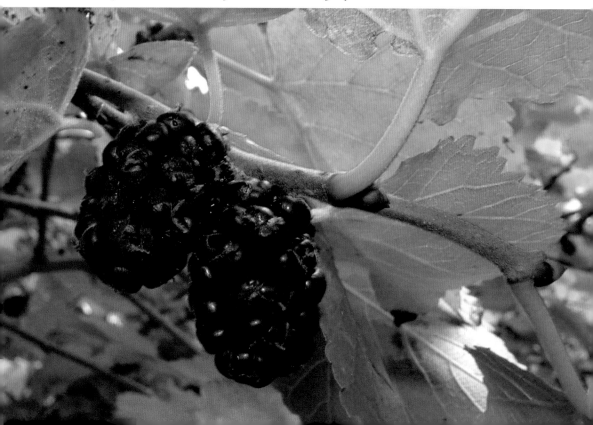

stuffing more fruit into his hood which is tied at the neck to make a bag. A man on the ground angrily waves a cudgel. Hoods of cherries are shown in several medieval pewter badges, but the significance is uncertain and open to many interpretations. One suggestion is that the badges represent good fortune and plenty. The *Cherry Tree Carol* tells how the Holy family are fleeing to Egypt to escape the wrath of King Herod. During their journey, Mary becomes hungry and spies a cherry tree laden with fruit. 'Joseph. Pray, pick me some cherries that I may eat.' Joseph, who in medieval times was often portrayed as a grumpy old man, who knows full-well that the child isn't his, turns around in a huff, saying, 'Huh! Let him who got you pregnant pick them for you!' At which God makes the cherry tree bend lower, so that Mary can pick some cherries herself. In reality, the tree would have been a date palm, and is sometimes shown as one in some manuscripts depicting the flight to Egypt. Maybe cherries were the most tempting and tastiest fruit that the songwriter knew of from personal experience.

Plums, bullace, *Prunus domestica sub. Sp. insititia*, and sloes, *Prunus spinosa*, are native to Britain. The stones of both have been found in archaeology dating back to the Neolithic period. Sloes tend to remain rather bitter, regardless of how long they are left to ripen. The fruits of the Bullace are larger than sloes and certainly preferable for modern tastes. Plums are rarely mentioned in medieval writings, except for when they have been dried, and known as prunes, which were often included in food recipes. Plum is often a generic term for any dried fruit.

One fruit that has been mostly forgotten over the centuries is that of the service tree, *Sorbus domestica*. It is very similar and related to the rowan or mountain ash, *Sorbus aucuparia*. The service tree was once thought to be native to Britain but is more likely to have been introduced into cultivation. There is a wild species in Britain, *Sorbus torminalis*. The small fruits must be left to blet like the medlar, or they have a tart flavour. The fruits are sometimes called chequers.

The strawberries of medieval Britain were the small, wild ones that grew on banks and in open woodland. The fruits are tiny, but full of flavour. Strawberries were one of the fruits that were eaten fresh, rather than cooked. Not everybody thought that strawberries were a treat; Abbess Hildegard wrote that strawberries were not good food for anybody, healthy or otherwise, because the fruits grow close to the soil and in putrid air. Strawberries were gathered from the countryside, but cultivated ones were available. Strawberry fairs were common. A mid-thirteenth century French song, *On Parole*, includes a tenor part based on the street cries of Paris:

Frese nouvele! Meure! Meure France!
Fresh strawberries! Blackberries! Wild Blackberries!

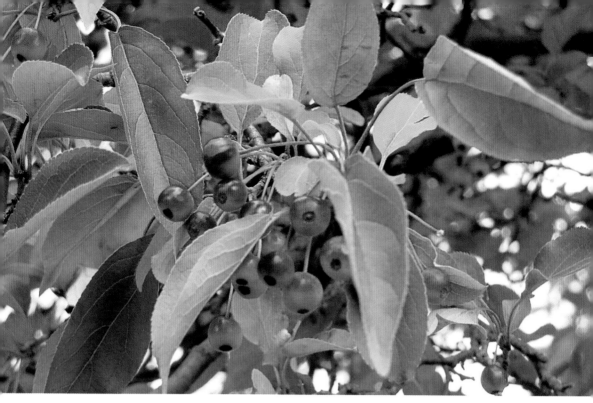

Above: Service tree fruits

Opposite: Strawberries were easy to collect from the countryside.

Unlike modern strawberries, the medieval strawberries would not require much labour to look after them and birds rarely eat them, so they do not need to be protected with netting.

The origins of other fruits that are now common is uncertain. Raspberries may be native to Britain but are not mentioned or commonly available until the early sixteenth century. Blackcurrants are likely to be native to Britain, but little is recorded of them as being used until after the medieval period. Gooseberries can be found growing wild, having escaped from gardens, but they are unlikely to be native to Britain. Gooseberries were being grown at the Tower of London, where they were cultivated for Edward I. Figs may have been grown in Britain during the medieval period, but were certainly being imported, most likely as dried fruit. One fruit that appears in medieval writings that would not have been widely grown in England is the pomegranate. The fruit could be imported easily enough, but it is unlikely that many trees grew in Britain. Friar Henry Daniel reported that he grew the pomegranate in his garden in London, but that he never had any fruit. He noted that the plant preferred as much sun as possible, but needed protection from any cold air, frost and snow. It is quite easy to keep a pomegranate alive in a mild climate or sheltered areas, but even today, the trees do not usually fruit in Britain because the autumn temperatures are rarely high enough.

MEDIEVAL PLANTS AND THEIR USES

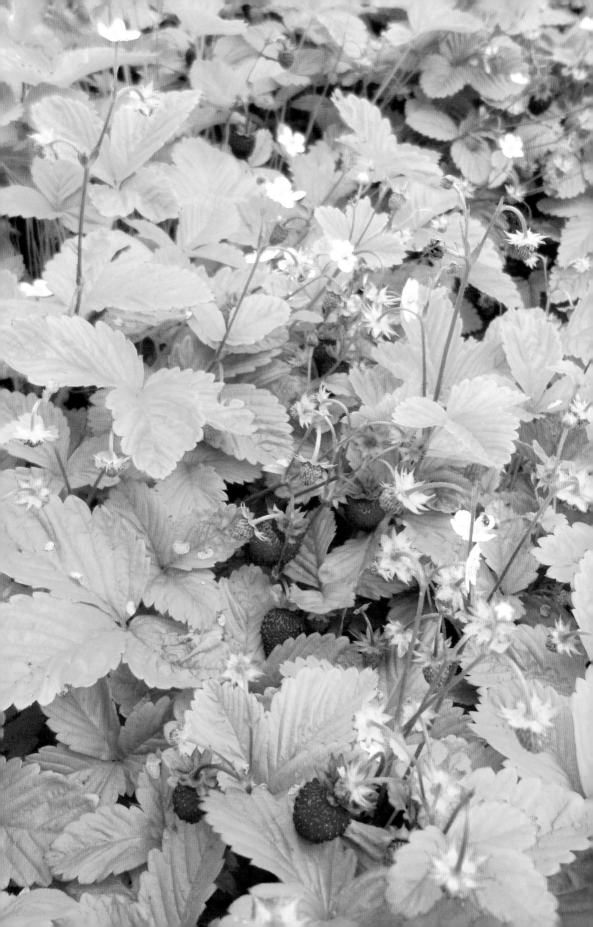

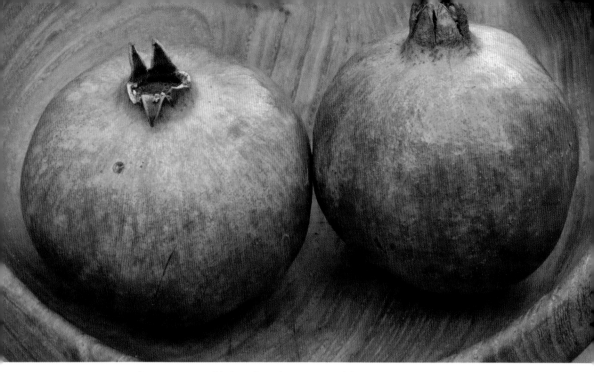

Pomegranate fruits were more likely to have been imported than grown in Britain.

Nuts are easy to store and provide protein and oil. Almonds are a major ingredient in recipes from the medieval times, and although it is possible to produce fruiting almonds in England, the crops are often poor. This would have little impact on the supply and use of almond nuts as they are recorded as being imported in great quantities. Almond milk features in many medieval recipes and with many people now drinking almond milk in preference to dairy, it is worth repeating a medieval recipe to show how simple the process is.

ALMOND MILK

Take almonds and parboil and remove the skins. Place them in a pestle and crush them, moistening with pure water then bring to the boil and simmer then allow to cool. The water used to boil onions and salt can be added if the almond milk is for cooking. The water can be strained through two layers of cloth and drunk with added sugar to taste.

Walnut trees were introduced to Britain. The production of nuts is not as good as on the continent, but the wood has always been highly prized. It was advisable not to sit under a walnut tree as they were reputed to give off noxious fumes. The convolutions of a walnut kernel were supposed to remind you of the human brain, so medicinally walnuts were used for treatments of the head. The outer casing that encloses the woody shell of the nut stains the hand black, making it useful for ink or as a dye.

MEDIEVAL PLANTS AND THEIR USES

Hazel nuts and filberts have similar properties. The trees can be coppiced regularly to produce wood, making them more profitable. Coppicing usually allows smaller plants to thrive in the brighter conditions once the hazels are cut back. The wood can be used for thatchers' spars and staples, wattle fencing, pea sticks and charcoal. The main problem with the nuts today is harvesting them before the squirrels get them first! Hazel can be left to grow as a small tree if you wish. If it becomes too tall, you can always cut it down to just above ground level and continue to coppice to keep it to the size you want.

Chestnuts are thought to have been introduced by the Romans. The tree will grow well in southern Britain, but the nuts rarely get to be as large as those grown in Europe, so most of the chestnuts that were eaten in Britain were imported. The wood has many uses. It is resistant to rotting, so it was especially useful for shingle roof-tiles, and fences. The nut was often included in recipes to make a stuffing for boar meat.

CHESTNUT RISSOLES

Cook the whole nuts over a low fire. Peel the kernels. mix together with hard boiled eggs and grated cheese to a paste and shape. Moisten with a small amount of egg white. Add powdered spices and damp salt and fry in oil. A sprinkling of sugar before serving is optional.

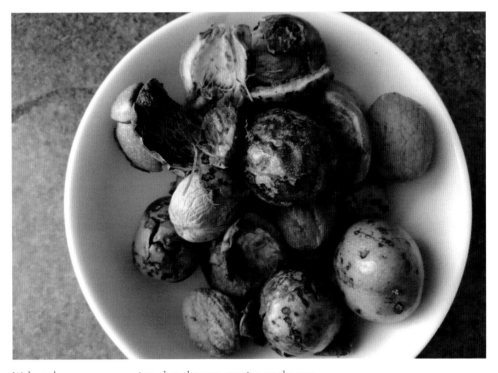

Walnuts have a green covering when they are growing on the tree.

CHAPTER 4

Grains

Grain crops were the mainstay for many estates, being a part of the crop rotation cycle. Grains provided ale and bread, essential for the B vitamins and calories at a time when everybody used more calories during the day as they were mostly more physically active than most people today and keeping warm in the colder months required a higher calorie intake. It is thought that up to eighty percent of an agricultural worker's ideal requirement of 5,000 calories per day would be provided by bread, ale and pottage.

All grains were used medicinally, with the flour of ground grains and bran often being used as hot poultices to draw out septic matter, and splinters of wood, metal, or bone.

Medieval crop fields would have been more colourful than today, with a myriad of other plants, field poppies, corn flowers, corn marigolds, corn cockles making a bright tapestry of colours amidst the gold of the ripening grains.

The corncockle with its purplish flowers was a noxious weed. The oil of its many seeds would not only make the flour rancid, but they were toxic too, giving rise to the plants medieval name, *Hell Corn*. By a strange quirk of fate, recent experiments have shown that wheat plants grow better in the presence of corncockles than they do in their absence! Although the toxic Corncockle seeds would spoil the flour and the bread, they had many medicinal uses and were considered to be hot and dry. Corncockle was often known as *Git* or *Gith*, the same common names that were given to *Nigella sativa*, an edible relative of the decorative flower Love-in-a-Mist; the black seeds of both plants are difficult to tell apart. Unlike corncockle, the seeds of Nigella are safe to eat, have a good flavour and are still used in many Middle Eastern recipes. It was the poisonous properties of the corncockle that Chaucer was referring to in the Canterbury Tales, when he had the Shipman accusing the parish priest of wanting to cause discord:

He would sow some difficulty
Or scatter cockles in our clean corn.

The stalks of older varieties of grains are much taller than modern ones and were used for thatching roofs, making baskets, bee skeps and hats, and for covering the floor

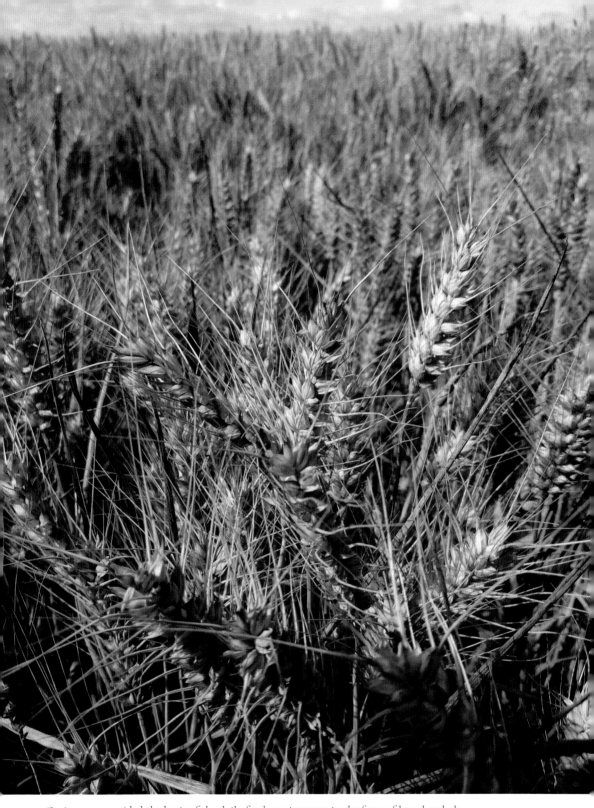

Grain crops provided the basis of the daily food requirements in the form of bread and ale.

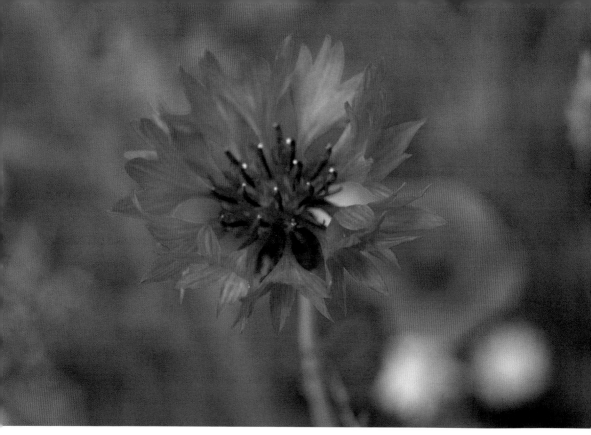

Above: Once common in cornfields, the cornflower is now mostly a garden plant.

Below: Corncockle was an unwanted common weed in early grain fields.

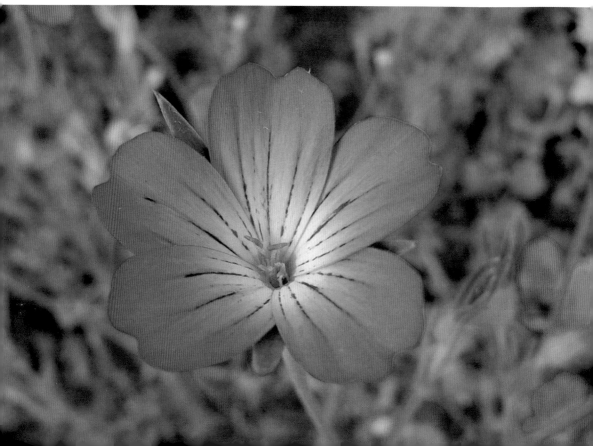

of stabled animals. Spelt wheat, *Triticum spelta*, continued to be grown during the medieval period. Spelt does not grow too tall, and usually remains upright, making for an easy harvest unlike Emmer wheat, which is tall and tends to fall, especially after heavy rains. Spelt has a lower gluten content than modern wheats, so the dough does not rise as high. Spelt-bread dough needs to be left to prove for longer than gluten-rich doughs or the bread will be very heavy. Spelt is becoming popular again because the lower gluten content is better for those with wheat allergies. It has a high vitamin B content and a good nutty flavour. Barley, *Hordus vulgare*, was used to make bread and ale. In the form of pearl barley, it was an ingredient of pottage and frumenty which could be served plain, sweet or savoury and was the ancestor of our modern Christmas pudding when it was made with fruits and meat. Frumenty can be served in a similar way to cous-cous.

FRUMENTY

Add one part of pearl barley to three parts of water, meat stock or milk and bring to the boil, then cover and simmer until soft. Check regularly to see if you may need more water. For a savoury frumenty you can add salt and a beaten egg. Sweet frumenty can be served with dried fruits, added as the frumenty is nearly cooked, so they take up some liquid. Drain excess water and add spices, cream and honey to taste.

Barley was used to produce ale, which was the most popular drink until the introduction of beer, which is ale with added hops that gave a bitter flavour and preserved the drink for longer than the usual few days that ale could be kept for. Ale came in two forms, small ale which had a low alcohol content and the strong ale, which was likely to make you drunk quickly. Both ales were made from malted grain. The harvested grain would be spread on the floor of the malting house and allowed to sprout. As the grain sprouts, it produces heat, so the grains must be turned, which keeps the temperature warm and even. The grains would then be dried in a warm oven. The grains were crushed and put into a mashing tub with hot water and left to soak and kept warm for about three hours to allow the starches to be converted into sugars before the liquid was drained off, allowed to cool and the yeast added. For small ales, the liquid may only be fermented for as little as a few hours before being drunk. The drink can be insipid, so plants such as costmary, *Tanacetum balsamita*, mugwort, *Artemisia vulgaris* and Ground Ivy, *Glechoma hederacea*, could be added for different flavours.

Small ale was drunk by children, women, clerics and the population at large. It provided vitamins and calories. Boiling made the water safe to drink and the alcohol preserved it for a few days. Strong ale was certainly available for festive

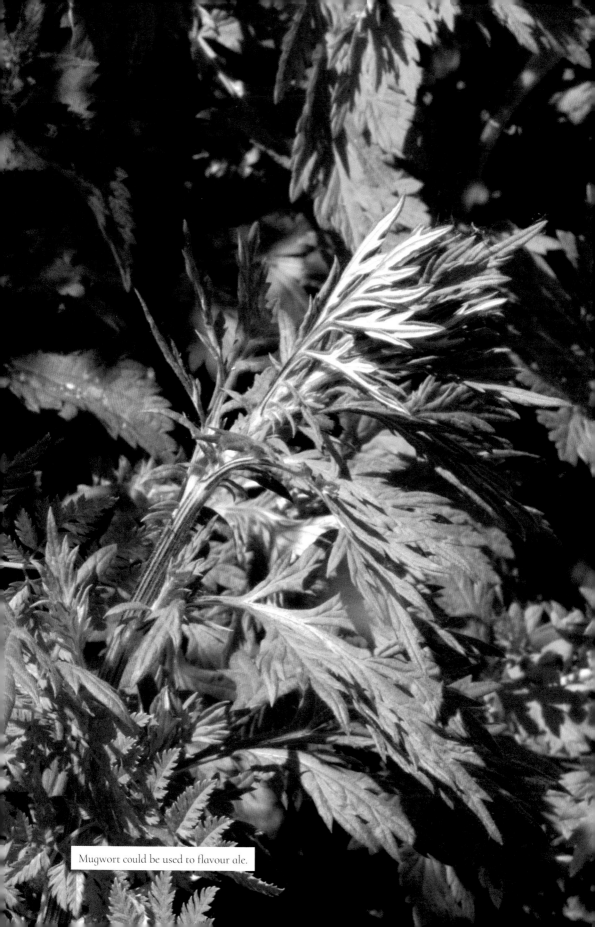

Mugwort could be used to flavour ale.

occasions. It must have been a potent drink because Bartholomew the Englishman wrote of three sorts of barley that were used to brew strong ale. He added a note of caution:

> Politicum, Dystichum and Nudum, of the which is brewed good drink and wholesome, whereof some so well like of the taste, that they drink three all-outs: the drink out of the pot, the wit out of their head, and all their money forth of their purse.

Oats were a good crop for colder climates and remained popular in northern England and Scotland. Oats were good for men and horses, although the bread was thought to be of very poor quality compared to wheat bread. Another grain crop was rye, *Secale cereale*, a tall, slow-growing plant. One deadly side effect of growing rye was the risk of ergot poisoning, often known as *Ignis Sacer*, or, St Anthony's Fire, which was caused by the parasite *Claviceps purpurea*, which became common on rye during wet weather. The effects of ergot poisoning included hallucinations, convulsions, erratic behaviour, or gangrene; death was common. Many of the side-effects are similar to those of LSD, which was first synthesised from compounds found in ergot by Albert Hofmann in 1938 when he was researching the medicinal uses of plants. Rye was not a common crop in medieval Britain, so the worse outbreaks tended to in be mainland Europe, although the fungus can affect barley and wheat. Rye bread has a very dark colour and being low in gluten, does not tend to rise as much as wheat bread, making it a filling meal.

CHAPTER 5

Plants and Medicine

Herbals

A herbal is a book of medical recipes that are mostly based on plant material, but may also include a wide range of animal and mineral ingredients. Some herbals included illustrations, but not all of them did. Most of the medieval herbals were based on those of the ancient writers of the medieval world's Golden Age, the Roman period, much as the Romans had referred back to the earlier Greek civilisation. Medieval scribes peered through rose-tinted spectacles back to a time when Europe was a united whole and scientific knowledge was at its peak. Following the fall of Rome, much of this knowledge was lost, or no longer widely available except to those who were literate, which usually meant the people who were connected to the church. The medieval writers initially took earlier herbals at face value, without questioning even the most obvious delusions and mistakes of previous writers. Many of the early myths about plants would continue to be repeated as fact into the Renaissance, regardless that they had been disproved by later authors. As the Muslim invaders of Europe became more settled, their scholars began to study and translate both Greek and Roman writings, often adding their own experience to the corpus of earlier knowledge. These volumes later became available to Christian society as the two conflicting cultures gradually began to trade, leading to an exchange of ideas and practical experience. Translations included the alleged works of Aristotle, although his writings on the properties of plants and their uses were lost. It was commonly thought during the medieval period that Aristotle was the originator of the theory of the four humours. Hippocrates, known as the Father of Medicine, was born on the Greek island of Kos. The collection of medical writings known as, *Corpus Hippocraticum*, is likely to contain only a few of the works of Hippocrates himself. It is possible that Hippocrates compiled the collection or part of it, but it is equally likely that later authors ascribed the collection to him as he was a respected classical authority. The ideas in the *Corpus Hippocraticum* include sound medical advice, such as assessing the age and bodily strength of the patient. The importance of a balanced diet and moderation was also stressed, which would become an important aspect of later medieval health care.

Dioscorides had been a surgeon in the army of Emperor Nero. He wrote *De Materia Medica*, which describes around six hundred plants, but also includes ingredients from minerals and animals. Unfortunately, the plant descriptions are often very brief or vague, which makes it difficult to be certain to which plant he is referring. Quotes from Dioscorides appear in many later herbals.

For more general information about the earlier uses of plants, we can refer to Gaius Plinius, usually referred to as Pliny the Elder, c.23-79, who was a contemporary of Dioscorides. Pliny wrote *Historia Naturalis*, a compendium on nature. This included a series of sections about trees and plants with their medical virtues and practical uses. Pliny was not very discerning about what he wrote, with the result that later generations continued to pass on the incredible tales and superstitions that he recorded. Having said that, his notes on cultivating vines were very practical and probably based on the methods used on his own estates.

The Arab influence on European knowledge began during the ninth and tenth centuries. The most famous – and most quoted – Arab writer was Ibn Sina, 980-1037, known to the West as Avicenna. To describe Avicenna as gifted would be an understatement. He appears to have had the advantage of a photographic memory, so that by the age of ten he had memorised the whole of the Qur'an and most of the Arabic poetry that he had read. At the age of thirteen he began to study medicine and had mastered the subject to such a degree that within a few years he was treating patients. Contrary to expectations, his *Book of Healing* was a scientific work, rather than medical, covering logic, the natural sciences, psychology, geometry, astronomy, arithmetic, and music. *The Canon of Medicine* was Avicenna's medical masterpiece and was often referred to by many later European writers. It is probably one of the most famous books in the history of early medicine.

Constantinus Africanus, 1020-1087, was an Arabic-speaking Christian who, having studied in the east, travelled to Salerno. Here he wrote books of his own and translated many Arabic works into Latin, such as Galen and Hippocrates. The *Leechbook of Bald*, written in Anglo-Saxon, dates to the early to mid-tenth century. This is the earliest known surviving European work that is written in the native tongue rather than Latin.

The first illustrated English herbal was the *Herbarium Apuleii Platonici*, written between 1000 and 1050; of which many copies were made. Following the Norman Conquest, most herbals continued to be written in Latin, although there were Norman-French and later, English documents. *Circa Instans* was one of the most famous herbals and influenced many writers. It was known by other names; *Liber Simplici Medicina*, and *Secreta Salernitana*. *Circa Instans* dates to the mid-twelfth century and is thought to have been compiled by Matthaeus Platearius at the medical school of Salerno, but this is debatable.

Later the book would develop into the *Tacuinum Sanitatis, Regimen Sanitatis Salernitanum*, of northern Italy. In English it would be known as the *Book of Simple*

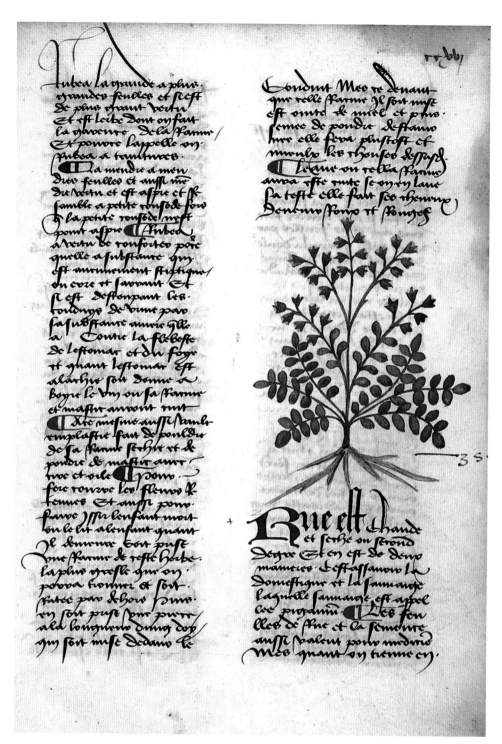

An illustrated page of *Circa Instans* showing Rue. (Wellcome Collection. Attribution 4.0 International (CC BY 4.0))

MEDIEVAL PLANTS AND THEIR USES

Medicines. This was a health book with medical guidance that was intended for the general population as much as the medical profession. Many copies were lavishly illustrated and show many interesting features of daily life, as well as the plants themselves. The book was very popular. There are two hundred and forty surviving manuscripts, with translations in several languages, including Dutch, Danish English, French, German, Hebrew, Italian and Serbian.

Many herbals were held in libraries that belonged to the church. The cathedral priories of Canterbury, Durham, and Rochester had copies of the herbal *Macer Floridus de Viribus Herabarum*. Many books were written by people of English origin. Norwich cathedral priory had two copies of the treatise, *De Proprietatibus Rerum* by Bartholomew de Glanville, sometimes known as Bartholomew the Englishman, 1200-1260. He wrote about gardening and the uses of the plants, with much of his information based on Pliny's writings but including some of his own observations.

Canterbury possessed a copy of another book written by a writer in England, Alexander Nequam, sometimes spelled as Neckham, who was Abbot of Cirencester in 1213. His *De Naturis Rerum* mentions about 140 plants, including trees and crops. The Latin text *Compendium Medicinae* by Gilbertus Anglicus, Gilbert the Englishman, was written around 1250. In the fifteenth century a scribe edited and rearranged the book and translated it into English.

Henry the Poet, c.1235-1313, described a square garden, set out as if it was within a cloister with about twenty-five plants on each of the sides. The plants all had medicinal uses. Another English writer was Henry Daniel, a Dominican friar living in England c. 1375, who referred to a garden that he once had at Stepney, London, where he grew two hundred and fifty-two different sorts of plants. John Garlande was an Englishman who was living in Paris during the thirteenth century. He tells us which herbs, vegetables and fruit trees he was growing in his garden in France. As he was in northern France, most of the plants he mentions would survive and thrive in most areas of Britain. By consulting the herbals and a wide range of other documents, including manor and abbey finance accounts, we have a good idea of the plants that were available and those that were being grown or imported for use in Britain in the medieval period.

Medical Theory

To understand the reasoning behind the medicinal use of the plants, it is necessary to understand the medical theories of the time. The body was thought to be made up of four liquids known as humours that reflect the four basic elements that were considered to constitute the physical universe. Each element had a quality; hot, cold, moist or dry. These elements were based to some extent on observation and were thought to balance each other in the real world. An imbalance could result in a natural catastrophe or at the personal level illness, and the fault generally lay with the patient. Hippocrates had divided people into a broad spectrum of four types of Temperaments, based on their personal predominate humour. The Temperaments were the effect of the humours on an individual. Their influence was the reason that you were an extrovert or an introvert. The humours were rarely in perfect balance in an individual; most people had a tendency towards only one of the humours. To remain healthy a person needed to keep each humour of their body in balance. The humours within the body were affected by the food a person ate, how their body processed it and the way they conducted their life. Each humour was thought to reside in a specific part of the body and predominated at certain times of the day: Blood at midnight; Phlegm in the morning; Choleric at noon; and Melancholic in the evening. The seasons of the year had to be considered too. Some authorities suggested where people lived, for example, a hot or cold climate, in the hills, on the plains or near the sea, would affect the temperament. Each race of peoples was thought to have a particular Temperament and even the different stages of life were related to the basic elements, humours and temperaments:

Element of Fire   Hot. Dry. Yellow Bile. Choleric. Gall Bladder. Summer.
Element of Water Cold. Wet. Phlegm. Phlegmatic. Lungs. Winter.
Element of Earth   Cold. Dry. Black Bile. Melancholic. Spleen. Autumn.
Element of Air   Hot. Wet. Blood. Sanguine. Liver. Spring.

According to Galen, animals, plants, and minerals had their own degree of heat, coldness, dryness or moistness. There are four degrees, of which one is the least potent. Lettuce was cold and moist to the third degree, so it was fairly cold and moist. Processing foodstuffs could alter their properties, whilst grape juice was cold in the third degree and dry in the second, the fragrant yellow wine made from the juice was considered to be warm and dry in the second degree, with the proviso that although it quenches the thirst, you should take care not to get drunk by eating something as you drink the wine.

Chaucer describes the Doctor of Physik as a person who:

Knew the cause of every malady,
Whether it was hot or cold, or moist or dry.

The skill of the physician was to keep the patient healthy by prescribing a good diet that would maintain the patient's balance of humours. If the patient was too hot, cooling foods could be introduced to temper the humour and make the patient well again. The patient had a responsibility to keep themselves healthy. To

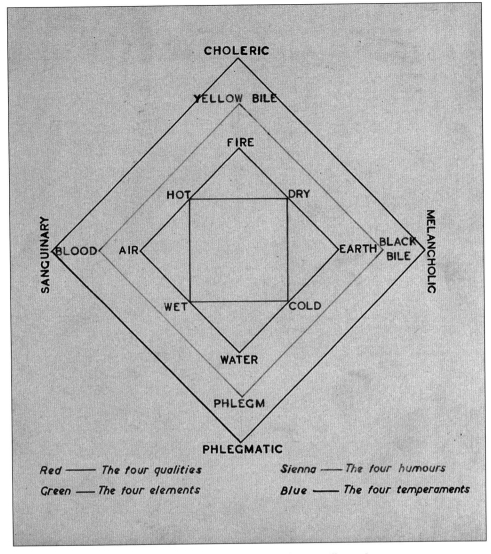

Chart showing the properties of the four humours. (The Wellcome Collection)

maintain health, nothing should be eaten or drunk to excess. Being on good terms with others reduced the likelihood of stress. Over exertion resulting from physical activities, including sex, was to be avoided if possible. You were advised to have adequate rest and sleep. Eating the correct food and exercising according to your personal temperament would maintain your health and if your humours became out of balance, putting you in ill-health, correcting the imbalance by adjusting your diet was preferable to purging and bleeding. Fish was thought to be cold and wet and would produce phlegm in your body. This could be countered by eating the fish with garlic, which was hot and dry, thus bringing the meal back into balance.

The main skill of the medical practitioner was in deciding whether to use a medicine made of one ingredient, known as a simple, or to balance the side effects of a more potent ingredient by mixing it with another that had the qualities to counter its extremes. If adjusting the diet failed to improve health, more drastic measures may be required. Excess of a humour could be balanced or removed through the body by purging, which tended to use toxic substances and plants, resulting in sweating, vomiting, urine, faeces, or tears. Snuff could be used to induce sneezing to clear the head. Coughing cleared the lungs.

A physician could save himself a lot of time by predicting whether the patient would live. A wounded man could be given a drink made with trefoil. If the patient vomited the liquid, they would certainly die. If the patient was suffering with the flux (dysentery), the physician should take an amount of town cress seed weighing a penny and mix it with water or wine. The patient should drink this for three days. If the flux ceased, they would live, with the help of other medicines. If the flux continued, the patient would die. If the patient was wounded, the doctor would prepare some trefoil for them to drink. If the patient cast it from their body, they would die. Slightly more bizarre, was to place greater celandine on the head of a patient. If they begin to sing with a loud voice, they would die, but if they began to cry, they would survive; whereas you would be inclined to expect the opposite. The physician could take a piece of vervain in his hand and ask the sick person, 'How do you feel?' If they replied, 'I am well,' then they would survive, but if they answered by saying nothing, or saying that they felt bad, then was little hope of them surviving.

For those who could not afford a physician, a local monastery may have been able to provide some medical care. For long-term care or for a terminal illness, it was sometimes possible to stay at a hospital. The medieval hospital provided care and comfort for the patient, but not necessarily the medical care needed to produce a cure. Leper hospitals were usually run by the church, with women to provide food and daily care. The church considered that illness was the result of the patient's sinfulness, and thus an act of God. To pay the sin the patient should suffer some form of penance. St Benedict had originally said that the care of a patient was one of the duties of a monk, but that curing them was in God's hands, not those of the monk! Although the Rule of St Benedict does say that, 'The use of herbs should be allowed to the sick as often as is desirable, but to the healthy and the young this should not be granted very often.'

So, if you were healed, you gave thanks to God and the saints, but if you died, God had willed it. Hopefully, you had lived a good life, and your place in heaven was assured.

By the first millennium monks were providing a wide range of medical care, but later the church placed restrictions on clerics practicing medicine.

The Diagnosis of Medical Problems and Ailments

Before considering treatment, it was essential to make the correct diagnosis of the ailment. How would the physician decide the best method to treat the patient? In a similar way to modern doctors, the medieval leech or physician would make a visual appraisal of the patient. Skin colour helped with a diagnosis for yellow or black choler, even if they did not understand what caused it. Urine could be checked using a glass jar called a Matula or a Jordan. Urine had the nickname, the Waters of Jordan! Ideally the urine was to be warm. The physician studied the urine for its clarity and colour, which could be compared to a colour chart, much like a paint colour chart, which would help the physician to assess the imbalance of humours to make a diagnosis. There may be particles floating in the urine. The smell and taste of the urine

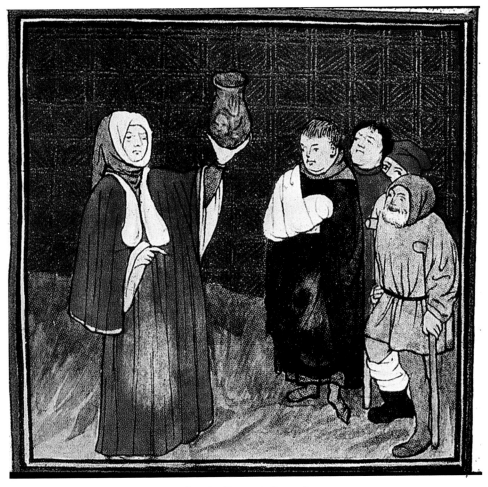

Physician examining urine using a Jordan. (Wellcome Collection)

was tested too. Testing urine was not a silly idea. Certain diseases do affect urine colour and blood would certainly show easily. A sweet taste would suggest diabetes and the smell can be affected too, as anybody who has eaten asparagus will be aware.

If the urine is red and gravelly it is caused by sickness in the kidneys.
If the urine is white and gravelly there is a stone in the bladder.

Astrology

The organs of the body related to different astrological signs and diagnosis used this as a basis on how to treat various problems. The physician would also want to know when the illness first began and under which astrological auspices this had been influenced. Treatment would be influenced by the timing of the cure. To ensure a

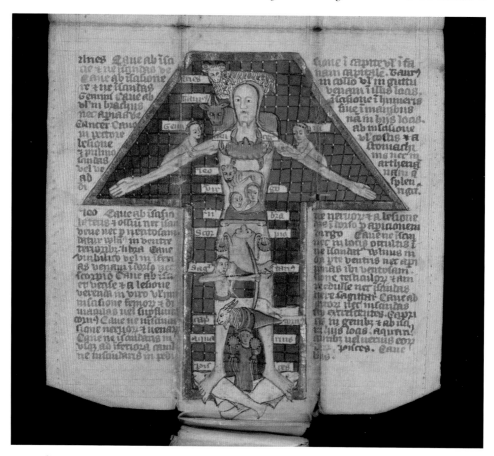

Pages of a Vade Mecum showing the astrological dominance of difference parts of the body. (The Wellcome Collection)

MEDIEVAL PLANTS AND THEIR USES

quick diagnosis, the physician would usually carry a *Vade Mecum* on his belt. This was a small booklet, with pages carefully folded several times so that it could include as much information as possible. A *Vade Mecum* usually included a diagram of the body showing the numerous bleeding points, astrological charts, and charts relating to the humours.

The skill of the physician was to use his knowledge of the humours, the temperament and age of the patient, the working of the body, diet and astrology to decide on the best cure. This could be something as simple as a change of diet or a medicine. Phlebotomy, the medical term for bleeding a patient, or purging were drastic measures to bring the humours back into balance. Sometimes the blood resulting from phlebotomy could be put to good use. John Arderne, a doctor who worked during Chaucer's lifetime, gave a recipe for an ointment called *Sanguis Veneris*. One of the ingredients that was necessary to include was the blood of a virgin maiden or a young damsel of about nineteen or twenty years old who has never been impregnated, because otherwise she would be corrupted. Finding such a maiden must have been difficult because Arderne complained that '... now in these times, virgins are seldom twenty years old!'

The physician also had to consider the best day to begin treatment. Certain days were auspicious, but many were considered to be very dangerous. These were the *Dies Nefastae*, the Evil Days. The dates themselves and the number of evil days vary depending on the text you consult. On Evil days it was best not to begin a journey for fear of never returning or suffering some misfortune. The Evil days were not ideal to take on a new business venture, nor to get married. Medically it was thought that anyone who was bled on these days would die or never recover their full strength

Month	Evil Days *Dies Nefestae*	Month	Evil Days *Dies Nefestae*
January	1. 2. 4. 5. 10. 11. 15.	July	15. 20.
February	1. 7. 10.	August	19. 20.
March	2. 11.	September	6. 7.
April	16. 21.	October	1. 6
May	6. 15. 20.	November	15. 19.
June	4. 7.	December	6. 7. 9.

If you had avoided the evil days and had been given a good medicine, you may still have needed to recite a prayer or a charm to ensure the remedy would be effective. Many of the magical charms are likely to have been pagan in origin and were later Christianised to make them more acceptable. The *Leech Book of Bald* is mostly based on English native plants with some classical references, but the cures often include the Christianising of pagan magical charms, in other words magic, but now it was Holy magic, so that was no longer a problem. Even in the fourteenth century, John Arderne, a more than capable medical man, would still recommend a charm to cure an ailment.

Nowadays the effectiveness of the placebo effect has been proved to assist a cure whether the patient believes it will work or not. A fake medicine can be as effective as a genuine one for many minor illnesses. If the patient believes that medical care is taking place, they may feel more positive of a recovery. Many medical problems will simply cure themselves, being resolved over time. Some of the herbs have properties that are still used by medicine today; aspirin was originally extracted from willow, and most over the counter painkillers are still opiate-based. Some plants had a reputation that it was impossible to live up to. Herbals claimed that betony would cure just about everything! It could be drunk as a cure-all tonic to keep you in good health. It cleansed septic wounds when used as a poultice. It would ease coughs, clear the eyes, restore hearing, clear poisons, and remove all filth from the body and cured the stone. Betony eased backache, headache, and toothache. It was claimed to prevent hangovers. Nobody should ever need to suffer again, as long as there was betony to be found!

Aches and pains and other common ailments

Having diagnosed the illness, the medieval physician now needed to know which particular plant would cure the malady that the patient was suffering from. One method of ascertaining the medicinal use of a plant was to study for clues from its appearance. According to the *Doctrine of Signatures*, God had very obligingly made many plants look like the medical problems that they cured. The small nodular roots of the lesser celandine were thought to resemble haemorrhoids, so that is what they would cure, whilst the flowers of birthwort, with their long tubular flowers leading to a round, hollow base obviously suggested the uterus and womb. Care may be required with the dose, as many plants that were used medicinally in the past are now classed as poisonous and considered dangerous to use. Some, such as mandrake, deadly nightshade and hemlock, were used to induce sleep. A milder and much safer sleeping draught was the root of valerian, a tall plant that can often be found growing in boggy soil near rivers and streams. It is still sold today for the same purpose.

One of the most poisonous plants was *Aconitum*, which was generally considered as too potent to be taken internally. Rue was known to expel poisons from the bowels, and was recommended to be taken internally, which is mostly considered inadvisable nowadays. Some remedies may have worked for slightly different reasons than those believed by the physician, other ingredients or the method itself being the important part of the treatment, not the herb that is specified.

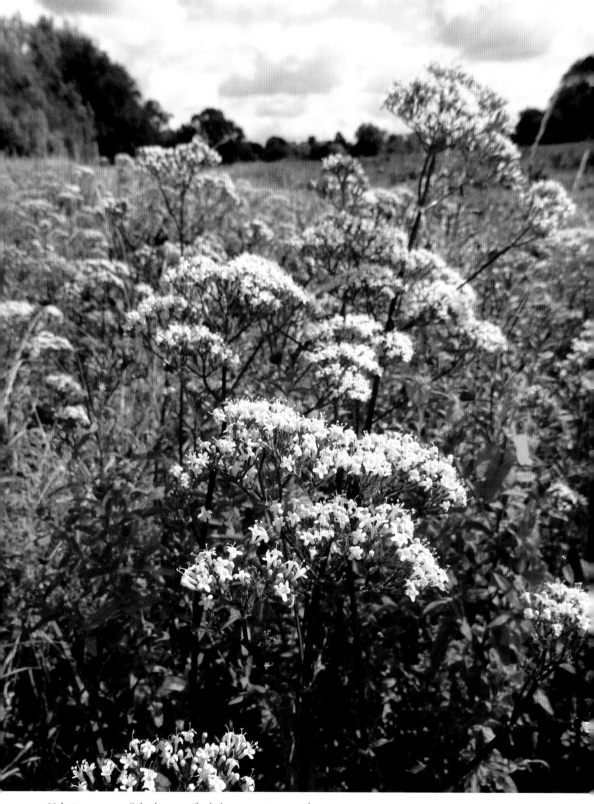

Valerian was a safe herb to use for helping a patient to sleep.

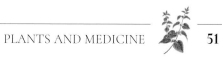

A cathartic medicine was one that purged the body, whether upward, or downward, and some purges were specifically used to induce sweating. Many of the plants used for purging were poisonous, so eating them exposed the patient to some risk. It was realised that an enema was probably a safer method to administer the purge mixture. To do this, the physician would use a clyster pipe to put liquids into the body through the anus. A wooden or metal syringe was used in later periods, but the earlier clyster pipes were made of a pig's or a castrated sheep's bladder attached to a wooden pipe. John Arderne wrote that the pipe was to be preferably of box or hazel, but if not, willow would do. The pipe should be smooth, well-oiled, and free of splinters and of six or seven inches in length, with a hole bored through the middle. He advised against using a pipe that also had holes in the sides, as his own experience had proved that his version was better. To use the clyster pipe, bladder should be filled with no more than a pint of the clyster, the technical term for the enema mixture, the thicker end of the pipe should then be put in the bladder and bound tightly. The other end of the pipe should be smeared with fresh pig's grease, butter, oil or honey, along with the physician's finger which should be inserted into the patient's anus and then the pipe should be slid in. Carefully pressing the bladder with the liquid between the hands would force the liquid into the body. Once the liquid was in, the patient should lie, 'grovelling', on the bed, pressing and rubbing their hand on the stomach, or somebody else could do this for them. The patient should force themselves to hold the clyster within them for as long as possible, but when they could no longer hold it, they could go to a seat with a basin beneath it, and 'there do their needs'. The physician would then examine the contents of the bowl for blood, putrid phlegm, worms, squiballiz (hard faeces), or pus, as this would help to decide which cures to use. The clyster pipes could also be used to provide nourishment for a patient who was unable to eat for some reason. If a person had no appetite to eat or drink then almond milk, pottage or anything similar could be put in a clyster pipe to feed them. Medical theory considered purging to be beneficial, whether constipated or not. People could be purged twice at least, or as much as three or four times a year with a clyster. Usually this would be twice in winter and once in spring after Lent, and once in summer; there may be more purging if the physician thought that this would be necessary.

Timing a process

In the days before accurate clocks, short periods of time were not easy to estimate when preparing medicines. Arderne used prayers that everybody would have memorised to help him gauge time, as in the following instructions. 'When it has boiled enough, take it from the fire and let it stand still without moving for the space of a Pater Noster, and an Ave Maria.' The Pater Noster was the Lord's Prayer and would have been recited in Latin.

Pater noster, qui es in caelis,
sanctificetur Nomen tuum.
Adveniat regnum tuum.
Fiat voluntas tua, sicut in caelo et in terra.
Panem nostrum quotidianum da nobis hodie,
et dimitte nobis debita nostra
sicut et nos dimittimus debitoribus nostris.
Et ne nos inducas in tentationem,
sed libera nos a malo,
Amen

A slightly more difficult method to estimate the time accurately was given in a recipe for a broken or open teat. You should take wood sorrel and wrap it in red cabbage leaves and then lay it under hot ashes for the time it takes to walk half a mile.

Cross contamination was a concern to earlier people who were making medicines. It was common practice to melt things in an oyster shell over hot coals or a candle. Oyster shells were cheap and plentiful, so it was no great hardship to throw them away. Tiles could be used in the same way. Egg shells were used as a rough guide to measure quantities. Nothing would be wasted as the shells were burned as an ingredient for some medicines and the white acted as a gum to hold other medicines together. The egg could be blown and rinsed out, then a liquid could be sucked into the shell, or for small amounts of a solid material, half an eggshell could be used as a measure. To measure the proportions of herbs to make the medicines, it was best to use scales with common coins as the counter-balance material, because to be legal tender they had to be of a definite weight; unless it was a forgery, or some devious crook had snipped the edges. A pennyweight was a common measure and readily available, unlike some of the higher denominations of coins.

Medicines

As with modern medicines, the treatments were used in many ways. A simple was the easiest medicine to make as it is made from only one plant product. It could be eaten fresh from the plant but was often boiled or simmered in water or wine. A simple of water could be distilled so that it would keep for longer. Simples were often added to other medicines.

An infusion could be made from leaves, stems, roots, seeds or flowers from one plant, or several, soaked in hot water, the same as making a cup of tea. The plant parts can be crushed with a mortar and pestle, then place them in a pan with some water or wine. A syrup, known as an electuary, could be stored so that it would be ready for use.

> ## TO MAKE A SYRUP
>
> Simmer the herbal ingredients, being especially careful when using flowers as they tend to lose strength and colour if they are boiled. Add an equal amount of honey or sugar to the infusion. Leave the mixture to stand for fifteen minutes. Heat the liquid to reduce it but be careful not to overheat as it should remain as a liquid when cooled. Store the syrup in jar with a secure top or a paper covering. If the syrup does cool as a solid, don't waste it, as it can still be used as a medicine. Syrups can be taken as they are or diluted with hot water and drunk. Take at breakfast time, and an hour's fast after, or three or four hours after supper.

The recipes often required that spring water or clear running water be used for mixing ingredients, although many liquid medicines were drunk in a good wine to avoid using water that may be contaminated. *Mulsa* was a medicine based on a quantity of honey mixed with a slightly less proportion of a decoction. *Pusa* or *Posca*, was a mixture of the herbs steeped in vinegar and water. Good vinegar rarely goes off, making it a good carrier for other ingredients. The water reduces the sting that vinegar can cause when placed on open wounds.

A lotion is a decoction that is applied to the skin. Many were simmered in water as required, although distilled waters keep reasonably well if needed in a hurry. They are applied by soaking a cloth in the liquid and bathing the skin. Lotions can be made using oils which keep better than water-based lotions. Olive oil was often the base for these medicines, but nut oils can be used instead. Oils were easy to prepare and had a good shelf-life compared to dried herbs as they are unaffected by damp conditions. They can be made using a simple or a compound medicine. There were several ways of making an oil medicine. You could bruise the herbs that you are using and put two or three handfuls in an earthenware pot or a glass vessel and cover them with oil. Seal the container with paper or a waxed cloth and leave in sun for two weeks. If the oil is too weak, you could warm it and press out the oil and add more herbs, repeating the process until the oil is the strength required, then it would be boiled until the water and juice had gone. Strain and keep in stoneware or glass vessel. A Cold Infused Oil is even easier.

Fill a jar with fresh herbs, cover them with oil and seal the top. Leave for two to six weeks. You may need to strain out the herbs and add fresh to obtain the desired strength. This is a good way to preserve Calendula and St John's Wort.

Ointments could be made of animal or bird grease; medieval recipes often specify which type of grease. Oil could be added to make the ointment softer, but there should be no water in the mixture.

TO MAKE AN OINTMENT

Bruise herbs and add two to three handfuls to half a pound of pig fat; vegetarian lard does work if you do not want to use animal fats. Pound the fat and herbs together in a mortar with a pestle. You can strain and add more herbs if you want a stronger ointment. Strain the fat into pots and seal. Label the pot. It should keep for a year. Small quantities of ointment could be kept in an earthenware finger-pot of clay sealed with linen tops smeared with grease or wax or by tying a piece wet sheep or pig's bladder and tying it in place. The bladder dries hard to form a secure top, much like a drumskin. To remove the top, you simply moistened the bladder to make it pliable once more. If you do not want to use animal fats, oil based ointments can be made by simmering the oil and herbs together. Strain the liquid and return to the heat. Add beeswax and stir. You can test a few drops on a plate. If the ointment is too hard, add more oil. If too soft add more wax.

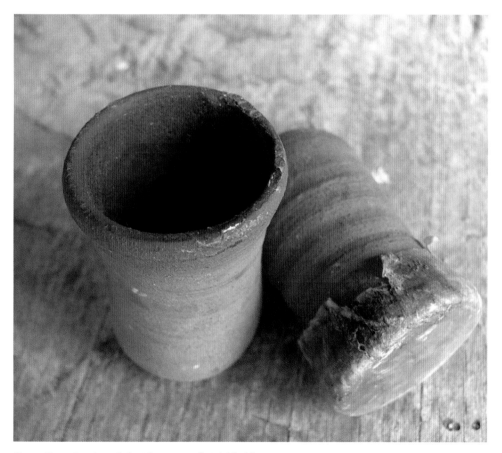

Finger Pots. One is sealed with a piece of pig's bladder.

Pessaries and suppositories were known as *colorynus* or *collyrium*, in early medicine. They can be made using animal fats or oil with wax.

> ## TO MAKE A COLORYNUS
>
> Simmer the herbs and strain them. Add enough fat or oil and beeswax to the liquid to mould to a smooth, cylindrical shape. The medicine can be inserted into the body through the anus, vulva or nostrils as needed.

Pills and Troches were another way of storing medicines. The ingredients may be the same for each, but pills were round or spherical, whereas troches were flat.

> ## TO MAKE PILLS OR TROCHES
>
> At night before bed take two drams of gum tragacanth and put half a quarter of the distilled herbal water that you need for use and cover. In the morning it will be a mucilage. Make the powder into a paste and shape. Dry in the shade and keep in a pot for use.

Herbals often refer to plaisters, which are poultices. They were generally based on fats or oils, or a combination of both, with the addition of the appropriate plant material and any other ingredients that may be required. The mix could be applied to a cloth and bound or placed on the body; sometimes plaisters were applied hot. Instead of using fat or oils, a plaister could be made of the herb material alone, or with some added honey. The plaisters to pull out thorns and other objects in the skin often included a cereal-based flour or bran. They were usually left in place for a few days. A plaister made of flour or bran would probably pull out the offending object regardless of the herbal ingredients.

Common Ailments and Cures

The names of some of the ailments may be different to the ones that we use now, but the medical problems themselves have not changed. Many of the individual plants were used to treat a wide variety of diseases, so a doctor or apothecary would need a book to consult to choose the most appropriate ingredients, as well as making a selection based on their past experience.

General aches and pains, bleeding wounds and headaches were as common in the past as they are today and would be treated fairly easily. Surgery was another matter, being beyond the scope of the herbalist, and the physician. Surgery was best avoided if possible, and was the domain of the professional army surgeon, or the barber surgeon. John Arderne stressed the importance of both the theoretical knowledge and practical experience of surgery techniques, when treating a patient.

Head Problems

The head can be afflicted by many ailments, but the most common problem of the head is the headache; for medieval people the *megrim*, a migraine, was the worst sort. Headache cures are quite prominent in the remedies. 'Chew the root of pellitory for three days,' suggests one remedy, by which time most headaches would have gone of their own accord!

If you could afford it, you could rub oil of mandrake on your forehead, which may also have sent you to sleep; or you could take mustard and rue and crush them together, add enough clean water to make a thick paste and lay it on your head. If your headache was a result of a hangover, henbane juice could be mixed in cold water and wiped on the forehead and throat. For headaches and fits, you could simmer the stems and leaves of wormwood in water, pour into a basin to cool a little then pour the liquid over your head to soak your hair, then make a garland of wormwood stems and wrap it on your head to hold in the warmth, and in a few hours

The roots of Pellitory-on-the-wall were a cure for headache.

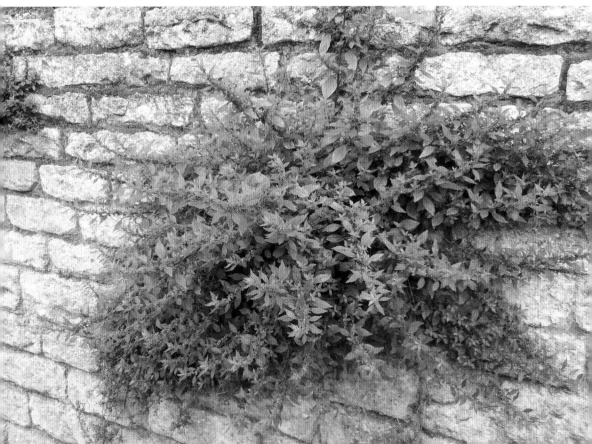

at most, you would be free of pain or so it was claimed! Slightly more toxic was a purge for the head that was made by mixing the juice of ivy with powdered pepper and then drinking it. Some head recipes were very general. 'For every problem of the head pound rue and mix it with vinegar and put it on the head.'

Alternatively, you could make a brew of 'betony, vervain, wormwood, celandine, waybread, rue, dwarf elder, sage and five peppercorns. Crush them together and mix with water and boil. Drink it whilst fasting.'

More pleasant was the following. 'Crush savin and mix it with oil of roses, then simmer and anoint the head with it whilst in the warmth of the sun during summer, or by the fire during the winter.'

Eye Problems

Because of the smoky rooms that people spent so much time in, there were many cases of poor vision, which was known as pin and web, a film covering the eye. It may have been Pterygium, sometimes called Surfer's Eye, Caligo, which is caused by a speck on the cornea, also causes dimming of the eyesight or simply a cataract. Surgery was possible, but there were alternative methods that could be safer, although experience was essential to not cause further damage to the eye. The greater celandine, *Chelidonium majus*, has a slightly caustic yellow sap that can cause blistering on the skin. This property was put to good use to remove the pin and web by dissolving the film that covered the eye. The juice was mixed with milk to temper its power. Pliny recounted that mother swallows put the juice of the greater celandine in the eyes of their young to improve their eyesight. This tale would be repeated for centuries to come. Putting caustic plants in the eye would be a risky procedure. Chaucer relates a proverb:

He that fully knows the herb
May safely put it on his eye.

If you didn't understand how to control the power of the plant, you could do more harm than good!

There were other plants that were used to improve the eyesight and were probably much safer for the patient. Meadow clary, *Salvia pratensis*, was often easily found in the local meadows. The clary part of the name is apparently being derived from the word 'clearly'. Eyebright, *Euphrasia officinalis*, is a semi-parasite that feeds from the roots of nearby grasses, Eyebright is a tiny plant that is difficult to cultivate, but if soil conditions are suitable, it will spread naturally in short grass or on exposed soil that is low in nutrients.

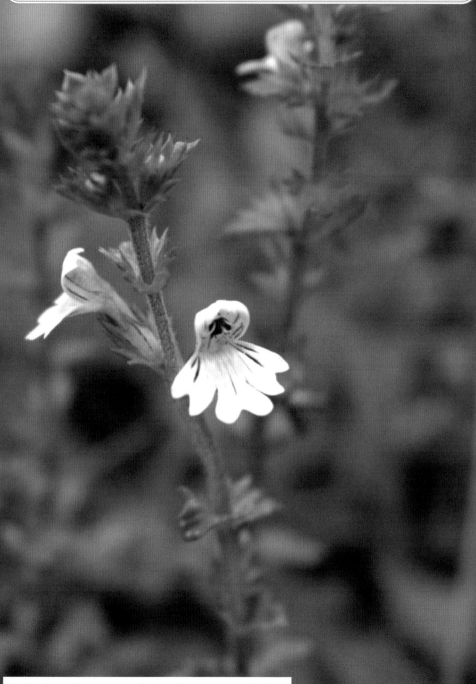

CONJUNCTIVITIS

Take eufrasia, known as eyebright, and pound it well in a mortar. Then pound red fennel and put the juices in a pan and heat them. Let it cool and put it in the eyes before going to bed.

Eyebright, *Euphrasia*, is a small plant that is easily overlooked.

> ## TO REMOVE WEB
> Take a good quantity of pimpernel, stamp it and wring the juice through a cloth. Take swine's grease and as much hen's grease and as much goose grease, melt them together and add the juice. Keep the ointment in boxes and anoint the eyes when you go to bed. Also, for this take a brass vessel and put in it the juice of woad and wormwood. Add strong vinegar. Leave it to stand a long time with a cover over the vessel. Put it in the eye when you need to do away with the web.

Nose

Problems of the nose could quickly affect other parts of the head, causing teeth to rot, the tongue to swell and damage to the brain, so they needed to be dealt with quickly. Depending on the diagnosis, a change of diet, no late suppers, care not to drink too much and not having too much sleep would be of benefit. A plaster of opium placed on the head was considered beneficial, whatever the cause of the problem. If the patient had a nosebleed, the physician should examine the colour and texture as this would guide his diagnosis. To stop a nosebleed, the recommendation was to insert the juice of betony, shepherd's purse or red nettles in the nostrils. To dry a runny nose, stuff the juice of mint and rue in the nostrils was used as often as needed.

Ears

Earache has many causes, with as many plant remedies to ease it. Worms carried the blame for many problems, including in the ears. Oil of the bay tree was poured into the ear which was blocked and left to soak for at least an hour. If there was a worm, it would now be dead and come out with the oil. If not, the juice of radishes was certain to kill the worm. Herbs were used to restore loss of hearing. In many cases the loss may have been due to wax in the ears, so the remedies may have been of some use by helping to loosen the wax. For aching ears or a loss of hearing, you could mix together equal quantities of radish juice and olive oil and pour it into the ears. The following recipe is more complicated:

Tinnitus, ringing in the ears or other noises, described by one herbal as 'similar to the sound of horns being blown', was thought to have many causes: bitterness of the mouth, heat and cold, or perhaps a viscous humour. A purge of choler was to be used if the cause was heat and of melancholy if the cause was from the cold. There were warnings of tempering medicines to reduce their power so they would not cause further damage to the ear.

Mouth

Stinking of the mouth and sores were the main problems. A purge to clear the stomach of toxic humours and a change of diet would solve much of the problem. Eating mint and spices would settle the stomach and make the breath smell pleasant. Treating sore gums and cleaning the teeth would improve the health of the mouth.

Teeth

Many things were thought to encourage corruption of the teeth and toothache. Choosing the correct diet would help, so to prevent teeth from aching, you should not eat freshwater fish, nor should you eat too many raw onions or leeks. Eating cold

The seed cases of Henbane resemble teeth on a jawbone.

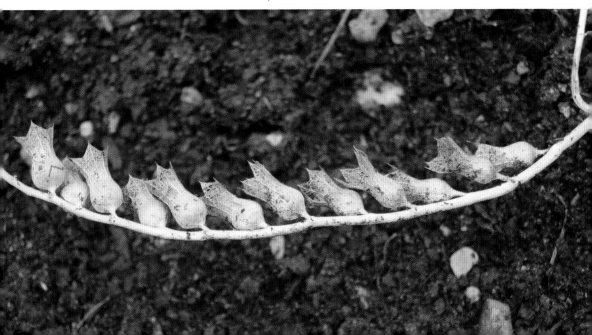

food soon after hot food, and vice versa, was also to be avoided if possible. Vomiting was another cause of tooth problems. The toothache itself was thought to be caused by a worm; the throbbing pain was caused as the worm wriggled and gnawed the root of your tooth. Kill the worm and the toothache would cease. The arrangement of the seed cases on the stem of henbane resembles teeth on a jawbone, so according to the Doctrine of Signatures, the plant must be good to kill the worms in the teeth. Inhaling the fumes of henbane seed would remain a common treatment for centuries. 'Lay henbane and leek seed with flour on a tile and heat them. Let the vapours reach the tooth and it will slay the worms and take away the ache.'

You could keep a supply of tablets ready to cure future problems of toothache:

TO CURE TOOTHACHE

Mix wild celery seed and a pennyweight of henbane leaves and two pennyweights of the avens seeds and grind them small with *Aqua Vitae* [brandy] and roll the mix between your hands to make small pellets the size of a vetch seed. When your tooth begins to ache, lay one pellet on the aching tooth and it will cease to ache in half an hour.'

The herbal adds, 'as has been proved'.

Throat

Scrofula is glandular swellings and a tendency to tuberculosis. The disease is characterised chiefly by chronic swelling of lymph nodes, particularly those of the neck, behind the ears, and under the chin. It was usually spread by unpasteurized milk from infected cows. It was often known as the King's Evil, as it was claimed that you would be cured if an anointed king simply touched you.

Skin

Accidental physical injury would have been a frequent occurrence in a society that relied heavily on manual labour. Agricultural work has always been dangerous, with accidents caused by animals, sharp tools and lifting heavy weights. Other trades have their own risks, including injuries from fire, boiling water and the side effects of handling dangerous materials or breathing-in poisonous substances. Personal injury from physical violence appears to have been common, without the added injuries of cuts, bruising and broken bones that resulted from warfare. There were many substances with antiseptic properties that were used to cleanse a wound and some are still used today. Wine and vinegar were used to wash wounds in preference to water, unless it was spring water which was more likely to be safe. Honey applied to a wound would cleanse and prevent dirt getting into the wound. Salt could be mixed with herbs to place on wounds, but it does sting.

Exterior cuts and wounds required a plant with styptic properties that would stop the bleeding, such as betony, the hedge and water Woundworts, or woad. Herb Robert was thought to be good for staunching wounds as the stems turn a bright blood-red in the autumn.

A herb that was known as a vulnerary, would help the wound to heal cleanly. Agrimony was a good treatment to ease and heal cuts of all causes, including sword wounds.

Thorns, splinters of wood or metal or pieces of broken bone could be treated with poultices which would usually work on their own, but other plants were usually included in the recipes, such as birthwort which was thought to be good for pulling thorns out of the flesh.

Apostumes, postumes or imposthumes were purulent swellings or abscesses. They could be defined by the colour of the skin around the wound and the liquids issuing from the wound, reflecting the humours of the body, Sanguine apostumes were red,

The red stems of Herb Robert suggested its use for staunching wounds.

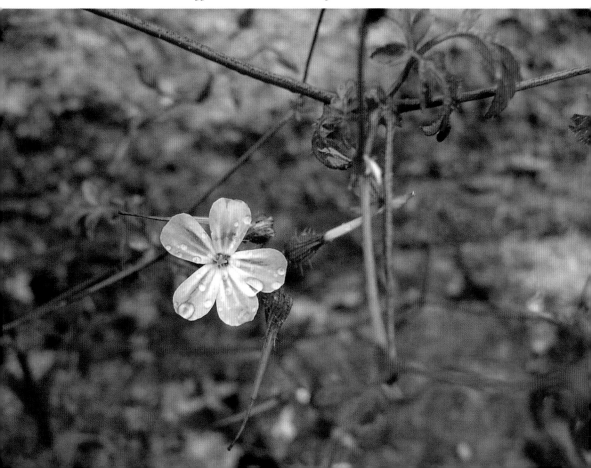

sore and throbbing; Choleric ones were yellow accompanied by pain and aches; Phlegmatic ones were pale and soft while melancholic ones were hard and dark, requiring softening to allow them to break and release the fluid.

Canker and Festers were thought to be the result of wounds that had not healed properly and had developed pus in the wound. This was usually because the wound had healed from the top, sealing in the gunge. The wound had to be broken open to let out the putrid matter in the wound.

CANKER WOUND

Take a drachm of hempseed and of rye and parch them on a pottery sherd until black. Add half a drachm of Verdigris and mix it with as much honey as is needed. Lay on the wound until the scab comes away. It heals both old and new cancerous sores.

For deep wounds which needed to heal from inside, the surgeon John Arderne provided a recipe for a valence that would keep the wound open to let it heal and allow pus to escape.

A VALENCE

Juice of wormwood, smallage, plantain and with swine's grease cleansed well of the skins, bruise it well and long in a mortar smiting it, but not breaking it utterly. And evermore put in a little of the juice to the grease that it may be well imbibed and that the tallow be made green. When this is done keep it for your use. This valence of wormwood helps bruising of the legs and shinbones, and to wounds that are made in the muscles of the arms and legs with a straight wound as of a knife or an arrow, or such other. And it helps all wounds to hold them open and it mitigates the aching. When you need to use it in wounds, add in two or three drops of oil of roses or of violets and anoint all the wound about and the limb that is hurt. Afterwards put in the valence on soft linen cloth and bind it completely and let it stay a natural day. This medicine represses swelling and aching and holds the wound open and draws out venom and eases the burning of the limbs.

Internal bleeding, whether caused by exterior physical force from a blow or fall or a medical problem was best dealt with without surgery if possible. Tansy and comfrey were easily found plants that were used to treat internal bleeding.

Chilblains, known as kibes, must have been common for many northern European people who worked outdoors in cold weather and when houses were much colder than

MEDIEVAL PLANTS AND THEIR USES

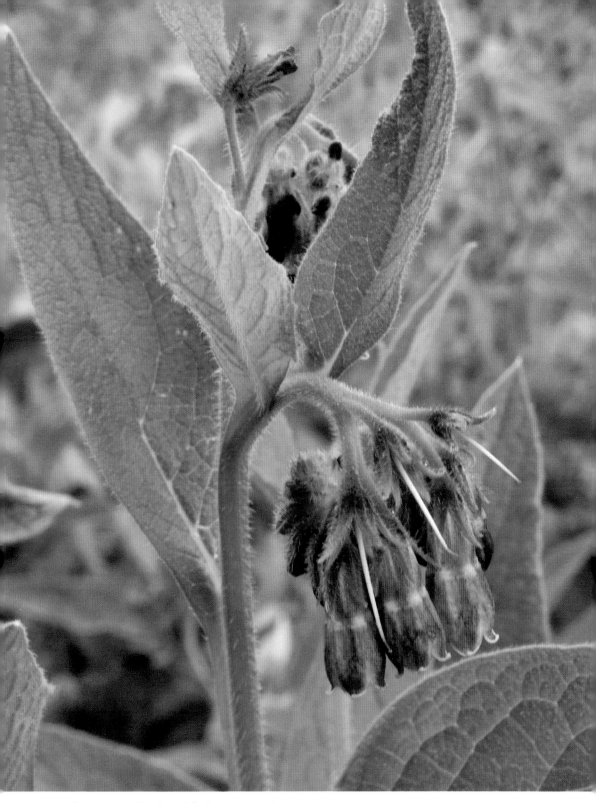

Comfrey was considered good for healing wounds.

 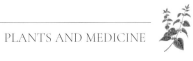

they are now. One herbal recommended treating chilblains with fennel mashed into eggs and wine.

One of the most feared diseases was leprosy. During the medieval period many people thought that catching the disease was the result of a sin that had been committed, making lepers social outcasts. Such was the fear of leprosy that lepers were isolated in special hospitals. At the time there was no cure for the disease, all that could be done was to relieve the suffering of the victims. Diagnosis was not always accurate, as many other unrelated skin problems appeared similar to leprosy and were often mistaken for it. To diagnose a leper, some of the patient's blood was placed in a vessel and some salt was mixed into the blood. If the person had leprosy, the salt would sink to the bottom. Once diagnosed with leprosy, a good ointment to ease the sores could be made of alum, cabbage leaves and sharp vinegar mashed together. Besides being suitable to abate leprosy, it would help other spots or rashes of the skin if applied regularly.

Jaundice

This is usually caused because of a problem with the liver, resulting in a build-up of the chemical bilirubin. The skin and the white of the eye become yellow in colour. Many of the early jaundice cures contained a yellow ingredient, referencing the Doctrine of Signatures. Most alleged cures were probably ineffective. 'Take the juice of yarrow and saffron and boil them in a sweet barley wort and let the patient drink it'. Another jaundice medicine that only the wealthy could afford, was easy to prepare.

JAUNDICE

Take an apple of the type that is called Red Steer or Ricardon and remove the core, then fill the hole with powdered saffron and powdered ivory. The patient was to eat one of these apples first thing in the morning and the last thing at night.

The Back

With manpower and physical hard labour being the main power source, sciatica, pain in the lower back and general back pain was common. Warm poultices were recommended. One such poultice included urine, the dregs of ale, wheat bran, salt, an ounce of stale breadcrumbs boiled together until they became a thick and then applied to the painful part.

Physical hard work in all weathers and the poor condition of housing led many people to suffer with arthritis. Hemlock is widespread plant and easily identified, so it would not be difficult for most people to make their own ointment of oil or animal fat and hemlock to bring relief.

Lungs and Breathing Problems

Breathing problems would have been common when rooms were often smoky. Dust would be a problem for agricultural workers working with hay and straw, especially during harvest and threshing. Fumes of varying toxicity would have affected many industries. The term *Asmaticus*, seems to have been applied to asthma and any other general shortness of breath.

Chinke, sometimes known as kink, kynge or chin cough, were terms applied to whooping cough or a persistent cough. The following remedy would help bring relief. Liquorice is still a common ingredient for modern cough medicines.

> ### COUGH MIXTURE
>
> Take four drachms of both clarified honey and May butter, an ounce of cumin, two ounces of anise, and three ounces of liquorice. Mix them together in the same manner of an electuary. Take when fasting.

The herbal said that this is a principal medicine and proved; or so the author insists.

To cure coughing spasms, eat Radish root or seed or drink Fennel Root in wine.

Liquorice root was good for coughs.

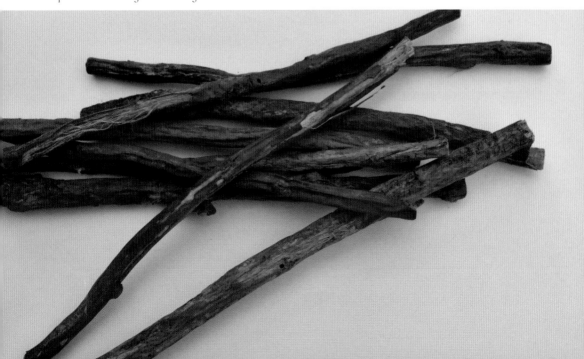

Hiccoughs

Yox was the name for hiccoughs, which are unpleasant and may cause embarrassment. Catmint drunk in wine would soon cure you. We don't know if people during the medieval period held their breath to cure hiccoughs or made people jump by making a loud noise behind them, but these are simple folk remedies that some people still use today.

A CONFECTION FOR THE CHEST

Take a quart of clarified honey, melt it on a fire and skim it. Be careful that the fire is easy and gentle, or the honey will turn black. Simmer it until it goes hard. To test this, drop a drop on a cold platter and it will soon go hard. When it will do so, mix in a pound of rye flour little by little until it is so thick it will not stir. Then let it cool. When it is cool, grind it into a powder with other such powders as you wish and strew the powder on a board. Then make a batter of bean flour and of wort (of ale?). Then take the seed of coriander, or of anise or dill, choose which of the three you will and put into the batter the weight of the seed you like. And lay it on the board with the powder. And roll the seed on the powder with a rolling pin until it is round. And as of the size of a pea or more as you wish. And this confection is good for the phlegm and for the breast.

Painkillers

Contrary to common belief, there were many medicines for pain relief that were available throughout the medieval period. Most were poisonous, such as deadly nightshade, hemlock, henbane, mandrake and opium poppy. In small doses the patient would remain awake, but often it was better for the patient to sleep through the worse of their suffering. One of the most reliable and powerful of the sleeping medicines was the opium poppy which was cold and dry to the first degree. The medical virtue of poppy was to bring sleep gently, but there was the warning to be careful, as an overdose could lead to the death of the patient. John Arderne advised that it was best to buy imported opium as the English climate was not ideal for producing a good quality poppy resin. Opium could be powdered and mixed with olive oil and sometimes rose oil, then rubbed on the forehead to cure pained eyes, and ease headaches and migraine. The herbals refer to three species of poppy, white, red and pink. The white flowered poppy was, and still is, considered to be the best. The method of extracting the opium had not changed until very recently. When the petals had fallen off, the soft seed heads were lightly cut to let the milky sap flow and then dry in the hot sun. Another method was to grind the seed heads to extract the liquid and dry it in the sun, although the resulting resin would not be so potent as the first method. A decoction of the opiate was given to the patient to give them an easy sleep, but if they were likely to die soon, it was better to wash the patient's face with the liquid to induce sleep and give relief from pain. It was well-known in the past, as it is today, that ingesting opiates could make you constipated. It was recommended that the patient should not drink, nor eat a lot of opiates at once, a pennyweight of the seeds at most. Any more could result in death, or at the very least, the patient may fall into a stupor. Another way to make an opiate medicine was to boil poppy heads in two parts of water, sieve the liquid, then add a third of honey. This would store easily and was recommended to be useful for many illnesses and to help bring sleep. The sweet honey would also mask the bitter flavour of the opium.

Arderne used poppy, along with other potent herbs, to make sleeping draughts to knock a patient out so that they would not feel any pain during an operation, or to give patient relief from the pain. He records that he would only use opium if he had added saffron to control the side effects. The risk of giving an overdose could be reduced by applying the medicine externally by mixing opium with oil of roses to anoint the patient's head. Mandrake could be used in a similar fashion. The juice of

the native wild lettuce was thought to be a much cheaper and was a more readily available alternative to opium. 'To induce sleep, mix lettuce seed with the milk of a woman carrying a daughter and the white of an egg and place the medicine on the temples.'

A febrifuge is a medicine to reduce a fever, of which there were many different types that were recognised by medieval medicine. Periodic fevers were named according to the time span that they recurred over. A tertian fever was one that recurred every third day. Symptoms included high fever, sweats, chills, and an aching body. A quartan fever occurs once

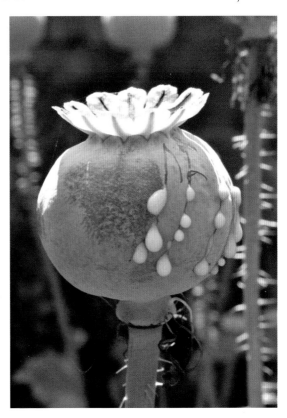

Opium was used as a powerful painkiller.

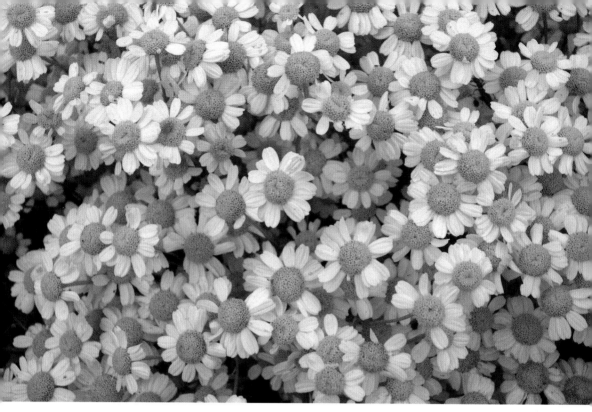

Feverfew was good for all kinds of fevers.

every four days and may be referred to as *Febris Quartana* in Latin. Quintana fever recurs once every five days and is probably what we call trench fever, whilst the quotidian fever is an intermittent fever recurring every day. The ague was most likely to be malaria or another intermittent fever.

Feverfew was good for fevers of all types and easily grown.

Bowel Problems

A large proportion of medieval medical advice concerned the bowels. Laxes, was a looseness of the bowels. A patient suffering from tenasmon would need to continually want to empty their bowels or bladder. Equally problematical was the flux, severe diarrhoea or dysentery. The bloody flux was dysentery with a bloody discharge.

One remedy for the bloody flux was to take flowers of elder and place them in vinegar for three hours then stamp them and leave to dry. A spoonful of wine or ale was then added. To keep it for later, it had to be kept dry.

If a patient was described as costive, it meant that they were suffering from serious constipation. Many of the purging plants would soon ensure that the patient would not have to suffer for much longer. Polypody, a fern that grows on walls or tree branches in wetter areas of Britain, was a common laxative, and if it was not very

MEDIEVAL PLANTS AND THEIR USES

effective, the prunes certainly would be! The violets, aniseed and fennel would make the medicine taste better.

> ### A MILD LAXATIVE
>
> Cook an ounce or two, or more, of the fern polypody crushed in water with prunes and violets. And add to it the seed of fennel and aniseed in great quantity and then let it cool. Give it to the patient in the morning and the evening.

Stomach-ache

The seeds of the wild celery, also known as smallage, could be chewed with some of the buds to help ease violent stomach pains and indigestion. Fennel seed mixed with the milk of a pregnant goat was recorded as being good for the stomach and freed constipation. The 'pain and twisting of the entrails that come from flatulence' could be eased by cooking cumin or maiden hair in wine with figs and fennel seed. Powdered calamint could be sprinkled on your food or drunk in wine to prevent stomach-ache or you may have preferred to drink wine in which you had soaked root shavings of a dried iris root.

Casting, that is, vomiting, your food may have resulted from many causes. Drinking an excess of strong ale or wine certainly results in drunkenness and its many side effects. Vomiting after eating food that was not fit for purpose must have been a frequent occurrence for the lower classes. Poisoning, intentional or otherwise, can cause vomiting as the body tries to expel dangerous substances. Another cause could be an underlying medical condition. To remove any poison from an aching stomach, you should wash fresh rue, mix it with wine and drink. And thus, according to the herbal, you shall be healed! Failing that, eating tansy, rue and southern wood with salt would probably cause you to vomit up poison or unhealthy food. A drink of mint leaves in warm water would help to settle an upset stomach if you were feeling queasy.

Intestinal Worms

Intestinal worms must have been common in the past judging by the numerous remedies that were recorded. The worm feeds on the nutrients that the patient ingests, and in a time of poor diet and times of famine, you couldn't afford to fatten a worm when you had little enough food for yourself. Worms in the intestines could be killed or expelled by using purgative plants. Most of the purging plants were effective in the main part because they are toxic, but they could be fatal to the patient too if the

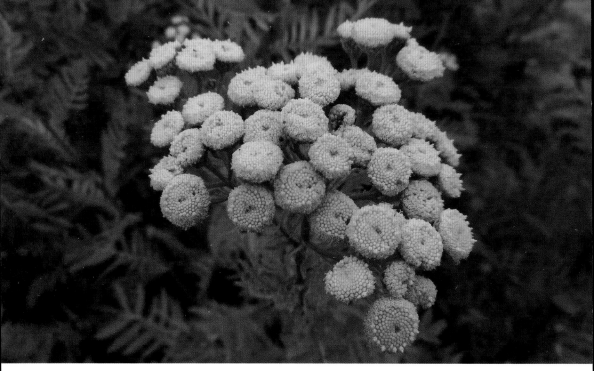

Tansy was used to expel intestinal worms form the body.

dosage was inaccurate. Wormwood, as the name suggests, could be made into a tea and drunk to remove intestinal worms. Other herbs with vermicide properties were tansy and centaury.

Urinary Problems

Stranguary was the name for the condition with the symptoms of slow and painful urine emissions. It is caused by muscular spasms of the urethra and bladder. A diuretic, a medicine to increase the flow of urine would be beneficial, so eating dandelions would be an easy solution for most people.

Stone. Gravel.

Both of these ailments are a result of a stone-like formation in the urinary tract due to a change in the acidity of the urine when a person is not drinking enough fluids, or because they have a poor diet. Most bladder stones form within the bladder, but some may initially form in the kidneys and then travel through the urinary system to the bladder. There were numerous recipes to break the stone or to encourage vigorous urination to help wash out the stones. Gromwell is a native plant of shady places. The greenish-white flowers are insignificant, but the white seeds have the appearance

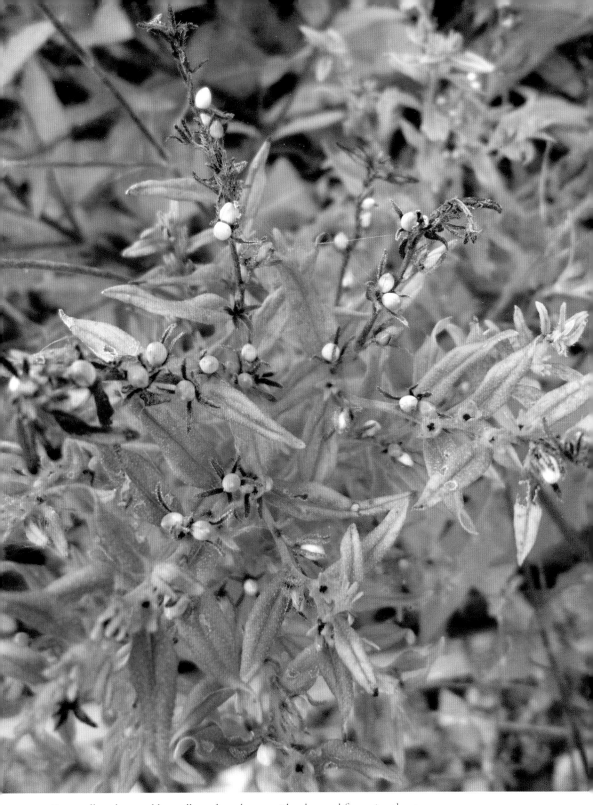

Gromwell seeds resemble small pearls and were said to be good for curing the stone.

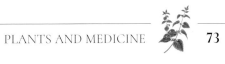

of small pearls and are very hard. Under the Doctrine of Signatures they resemble stones, so were used to cure the stone. The citrus-scented southernwood could be taken for stones in the kidneys but was also good for gout and fevers.

Plague and pestilence were general terms for any deadly disease affecting most of the population, and there were many such plagues The most famous plague, the Black Death, was simply known as the Great Pestilence, when it originally began.

The real cause of the plague was not known during the medieval period. Usually, bad air was blamed. You were advised to keep the windows on the south side of a building closed as the south wind was thought to be pestilential. Opening the north windows would allow a beneficial fresh air to clear the bad airs and odours from the house. For personal cleanliness you were advised to wash your mouth, face, eyes and hands with rosewater mixed with vinegar. If you could not obtain rosewater, strong vinegar would be fine, and it was a good cleansing fluid for all surfaces.

Bites and Stings

The bites and stings of insects and venomous beasts could be a serious problem. The 'venomous beasts' of the herbals included scorpions and poisonous spiders, but bites from these were not something that most British people would have had needed to fret over. In the days before modern treatments, bites, especially those that became infected, could prove fatal. Snake bites were often mentioned, especially those of the adder. Many plants were suggested as being a reliable antidote to a variety of bites, including pulverised leeks. In reality these cures probably worked as much by default, as a young, healthy adult should survive the bite of an adder unless they have an underlying medical condition that makes them susceptible to the venom. The greatest worry would be to the patient themselves and their family. If a physician could be seen to be taking any positive action to provide a cure, it would at the least reassure everybody.

With its association with the Virgin Mary, the Madonna Lily was thought to be such a pure plant that drinking the juice mixed in wine would cure a snakebite. Alternatively, you could apply lily pulp on the place where the snake had bitten you.

From the number of treatments offered in the herbals, a common worry for many people during earlier and medieval times was the bite of a mad dog. The bite of mad dogs was most likely referring to rabid dogs, although a bite from even a healthy dog is likely to cause infection and become septic. Any dog bite is best dealt with quickly to avoid complications. Vinegar, salt and honey would usually be close to hand for cleaning and sterilising the wound. Most of the herbs listed as being good for dog bites may have helped cleanse a septic bite but would have been totally ineffective against rabies.

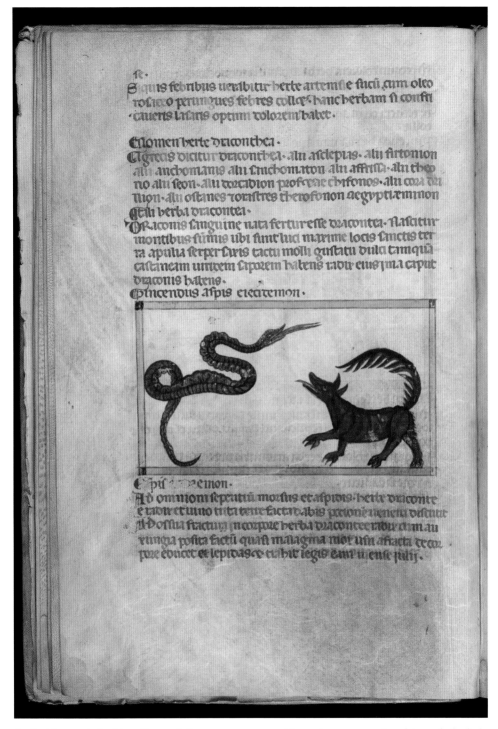

Ɍ·

Siquis febribus uexabitur herte artemise suci cum oleo rosaceo perunques febres colleꝯ hanc herbam si confricauens lasans optimū doloꝛem habet·

Ellomen herte dracontea·

Agrecis dicitur dracontea· alii asclepias· alii sirtonion alii anchomanis alii cinchomaton· alii affrisa· alii theono alii seon· alii dorcidion profecae chisonos· alii coꝛa dꝛ lion· alii ostanes toristres therofonon aegyptiæ minon Stii herba drancontea·

Dracoms sanguine nata fertur esse dracontea· Nascitur montibus sūmis ubi sunt luci maxime locis sanctis terra apulia serper suris tactu molli gustatu dulci tamquā castaneam uimitem saporem habens radix eius ima caput draconis habens·

Jncendius aspis electemon·

Chis demon·

Ad omnium serpentiū morsus et aspidis· herta draconte e radit et uino tita bene facta dabis poaoné uenenū distitur Al ossua fractura incorpore herba dracontea radix cum aurunga posita facta quasi malagma mor usu afracta recorpore educet et lepidas ꝗ eiabit legis eam u ense iulij·

Snake bites and the bite of a mad dog are common problems that are mentioned in early herbals. (The Wellcome Institute)

Haemorrhoids are commonly known as piles. There were many cures for piles. The tuberous roots of the lesser celandine have a similarity of shape to haemorrhoids, so according to the Doctrine of Signatures, they would cure them. A simple ointment of the roots pulverised in a fat would suffice. Later in the year it would be easier to find the common weed, *Galium aparine*, which has many common names including, goosegrass, cleavers and Sticky Willie.

FOR PILES

Take an unseeded leek and the herb that is called cleavers, that young geese eat. Put them in a mortar with some May butter and pound together. Lay on a linen cloth and heat them by a fire as hot as the sick person can stand. Place on the fundament and bind in place so it will not fall off. And he shall be eased in three or four days.

Slightly more painful, pulverise a handful of mullein with a pestle and mortar and put it in a vessel with olive oil and old boar's grease and boil them together, stirring well. Lay the mix on a cloth and apply to the fundament, as hot as the patient will suffer. And do this regularly until the piles are driven back in.

A different tactic again used mullein, but this time as smoke. 'Take a pan with hot coals in it and place the dried leaves of the herb that is called mullein. Put the pan under a chair or a commode, so that the smoke may ascend to the fundament, as hot as you can stand.'

The roots of the lesser celandine resemble haemorrhoids.

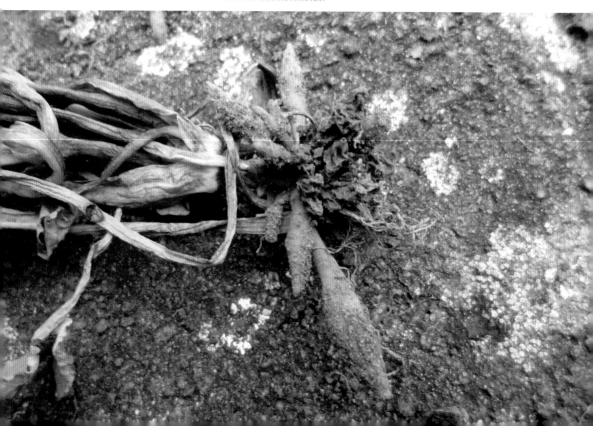

If illness and life in general was getting you down, and you needed a good tonic that would make things more bearable, a distillation of borage was to be taken as often as you liked. It would make you light-hearted and merry of good cheer. It was good for the blood and was worth taking if you were recovering from any illness. The root was the best part of the plant to use, then the seed. The leaves were only to be used if they were fresh.

Borage was a good tonic.

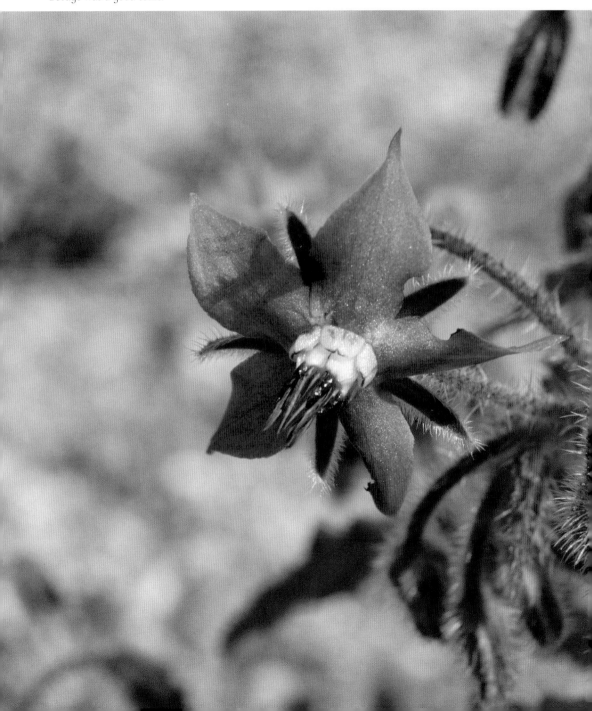

CHAPTER 6

Symbolism and Superstition

Plants, whether commonly known ones or not, inspired stories and gathered their own symbolism. On the third day of creation, God divided the land from the seas and carpeted the land with vegetation. Adam was to tend the Garden of Eden until he and Eve were forced to leave. For Christians, sweetly scented or pretty plants were invariably associated with the Virgin Mary. Poisonous plants were deemed to be used by witches for evil purposes and the works of the devil, even though most of them were used beneficially to treat patients. Sometimes plants were used to illustrate a moral point, such as when the medieval monk Strabo wrote that sage was a useful plant that could be used to treat many ailments, but you must cut away all the new growth or it will strangle the older wood. He was emphasising the common belief that older things were better and more stable, than new-fangled ones, although most modern gardeners would actually prune out the old wood to keep the plant as young and vigorous as possible.

For medieval people, the rose was the most highly favoured flower. Strabo said roses represented the martyrs and war, whilst lilies were for peace, although for many people in modern times it is lilies that suggest funerals. Roses can be seen in tapestries, manuscript illuminations, embroidery, carvings, stained glass, and they are mentioned in many medieval stories, poems and songs. The rose was the most perfect flower of them all. The *Macer Herbal* proclaims that 'The rose is the flower of all flowers as she over-passes all other flowers in scent, character and manner.'

The Eleanor Cross at Geddington, Northamptonshire has many roses carved on it. Maybe the sorrowful Edward I wanted the roses to demonstrate that his late wife had surpassed all other women.

The clerics at York Minster had similar thoughts, as just inside the entrance of the Chapter House there is an inscription painted in gold letters on a red background, *Ut rosa flos florum, sic est domus ista domorum* 'as the rose is the flower of flowers, so this is the house of houses'.

Yet initially the church had wanted nothing to do with the rose. Its association with decadent roman orgies, imagined or otherwise, and the pagan goddesses of carnal love, meant that the rose was as sinful as a flower could possibly be. But everybody loved roses and the church soon found a way to make the rose its own, so that it

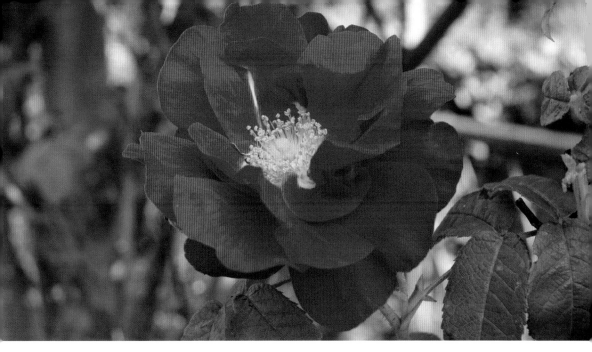

Initially the church frowned on roses, but later took them into its fold.

was not long before both the red and white roses had become assimilated into the company of God. For the church, the red rose was also the blood of the martyrs, and the most perfect martyr was Christ himself. The white rose was symbolic of purity and there was nobody on earth who was purer or more without blemish than the Blessed Virgin Mary, the mother of Christ. In his vision of heaven, Dante wrote of a vision of paradise, where Mary, the Queen of Heaven is the white rose bathing in the bright light of the sun that represented God and Christ. Because of the Immaculate Conception, Mary was also, *Rosa Sine Spinis*, the Rose without Thorns. Some traditions say that the roses that grew in the Garden of Eden had no thorns and that thorns only appeared after the Fall and expulsion from Eden. Mary and the baby Jesus were often depicted in beautiful gardens filled with the colour, bathed in the scent of red and white roses, both roses having religious symbolism. The five petals of the simple red rose are the five wounds that Christ received at his crucifixion. They were Five Joys of Mary: The Annunciation, Nativity, Resurrection, Ascension, and Assumption. The number of Mary's Joys has varied and mostly they are now said to be seven in number. Mary's name in Latin is Maria, each of the five letters of her name represented by a rose petal. The garden that Mary resided in was known as a rosary and may have inspired the idea of rosary beads to aid prayer and meditation. Beads had been used for religious purposes for millennia, but their use with Christian devotion is attributed to St Anthony the Great, or St Pachomius the Great in the fourth century.

The idea of rosary beads being originally made of rose petals is dubious. Beads can be made using rose petals, but their use is not recorded from the medieval period, and they do not seem to have become popular until the early twentieth century.

ROSE PETAL BEADS

Collect the rose petals and tear off the white parts of the petals and throw them away. The white part does not break down properly and will cause the beads to fall apart, as I discovered to my cost when I failed to remove them. Pound the petals with a pestle and mortar then roll the pulp into balls and dry them on a wooden skewer in the sun. You can string the beads once they are fully dry. Extra rose oil will be needed to give the beads a stronger scent. It is a fun experiment if nothing else.

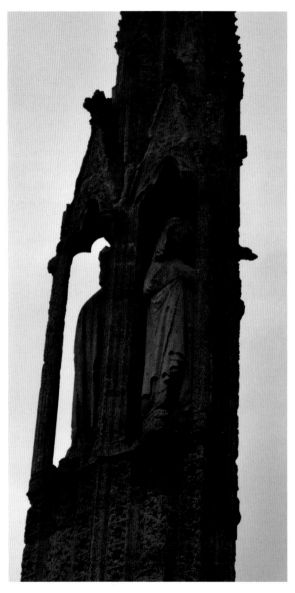

A friend threaded fresh rose buds onto a cord using a sewing needle. The cords were hung to dry and worn as bracelets or necklaces. They do not have a long life if worn regularly, but they were pretty while they lasted.

The poets who wrote of Romantic Love changed the religious symbolism of the red rose on its head so that it now came to represent the perfect woman who was the subject of the poet's words and desires. Plant symbolism was assimilated into heraldry and national and family traditions. Scotland chose the thistle as its national plant, and Wales the leek. With a sense of superiority, England chose the rose, but when the idea came about is hard to say. A monk of St Marys Abbey, York in 1368 noted that the 'Red Rose is the badge of England and has grown in this country for as long as man goeth.'

Roses feature prominently in the carvings at Geddington's Eleanor Cross.

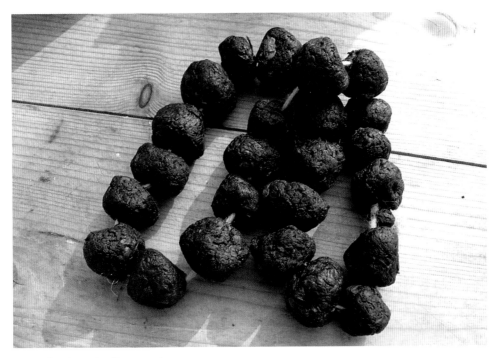

Rosary beads made of rose petals.

But the native roses of England are pink or white. The red rose, the Apothecary Rose, was certainly introduced and may not have been growing in England for such a lengthy period before the above comment had been made.

Not all roses were pure. Rosamund Clifford, The Fair Rosamunde, was the beautiful mistress with whom Henry II dallied when he was away from his wife, queen Eleanor. There are legends that Eleanor gave Rosamund the choice of dying by poison or a dagger, but in reality, Rosamund survived to retire to Godstow Abbey, near Oxford, where she was buried close to the altar. Her tomb at Godstow Priory was said to bear the inscription,

> *Hic jacet in tumba Rosa Mundi, non Rosa munda,*
> *Non redolet, sed olet, quae redolere solet.*

> Here rests Rosamund, but she was not a chaste rose,
> The smell that rises from her now is not the scent of roses.

Although one document adds the words:

> *Adorent, utque tibi detur requies Rosamunda precamur.*
> Let them adore...and we pray that rest be given to you, Rosamund.

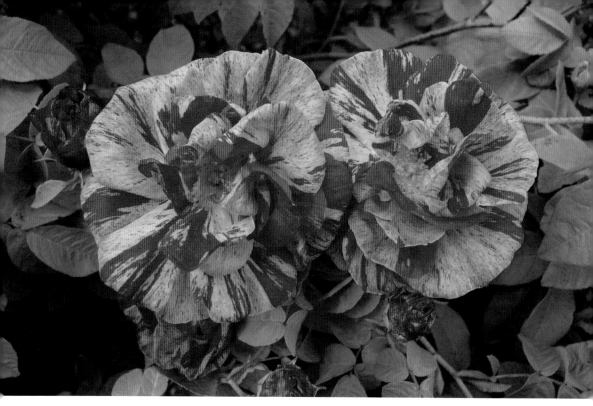
Rosamundi was unlikely to have been flowering during medieval times.

There is a rose that is a naturally arising Variant of the red gallica rose, known as Rosamundi, that has petals that are a swirling mix of a pink-red colour and white. The rose is said to have been named after the Fair Rosamund. Unfortunately, although it is a good story, the rose is not shown in any medieval manuscripts and it is not even mentioned in England until around 1653 by Thomas Hanmer, when he says it is a rare plant that was first discovered growing from a red rose in Norfolk a few years previously.

Roses were not all about status or romance, they also provided a little fun. There is a medieval verse riddle that is about the *aestivation*, the way that sepals and petals are arranged around the flower bud, of the dog rose, *Rosa canina*:

Qunique sumus frateres, et eodem tempore nati
Sunt duo barbate, duo sunt barba absque create
Unus et e quinque non est barbatus utrinque.

The Five Brothers of the Rose
On a summer's day, in sultry weather,
Five brethren were born together.
Two had beards and two had none,
And the other had but half a one.

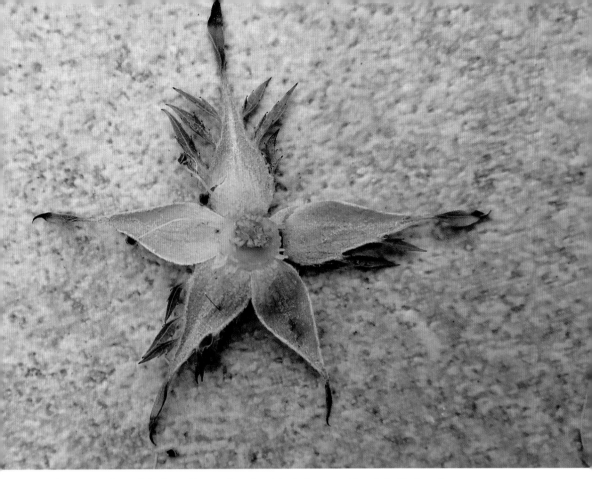

The Five Brothers of the Rose. The sepal on the right is the one with only half a beard.

If you examine the sepals of a dog rose, two of the sepals have smooth sides, two have serrated, or bearded sides, and the remaining sepal has one side that is smooth, and the other is serrated.

This idea of the rose being the peak of perfection along with the idea of the five sepals protecting the valuable petals may have inspired John of Gaddesden in the fourteenth century to name his newly completed medical treatise, which is made up of five sections, *Rosa Medicinae*. He described how he came to choose the title of his book: '...and I have so called it, on account of five appendages which belong to the rose, as it were five fingers holding it, concerning which it is written.' With no false modesty, he continued to say that as the rose excels all flowers, so his book excelled all other treatises on the practice of medicine!

Not to be outdone, Bernard Gordon, who had begun teaching in 1285 at the Montpellier medical school, completed his own book in 1305. He named it after the flower that he thought was the best, the lily, so his book was *Lilium Medicinae*. It quickly became such a popular medical book that Henry V's physician, Nicholas Colnet, left his personal copy to Exeter cathedral in his will.

Roses were more than beautiful and symbolic. They provided oils and waters that were used in medicines, cosmetics, food flavourings, and for potpourri and pomanders. Roses were considered suitable as a payment for the rent of land, as were spices such as pepper and cumin.

The rose was not the only flower to be associated with love. The delicate cerulean blue flowers of forget-me-nots were worn or given as tokens of love. The French

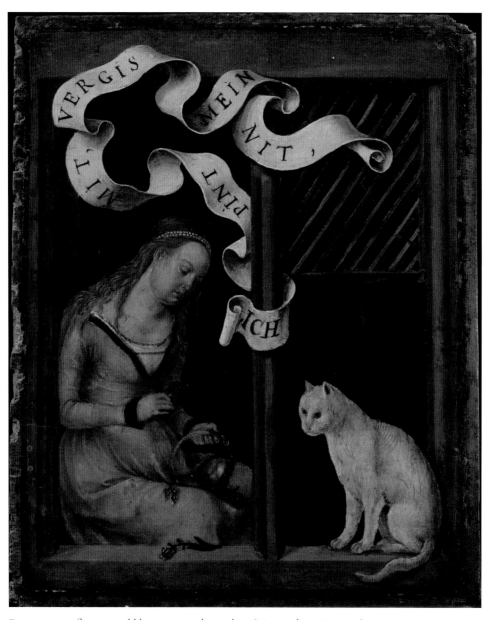

Forget-me-not flowers could be given as a love token. (Metropolitan Museum)

MEDIEVAL PLANTS AND THEIR USES

knew the flowers as, *ne m'oubliez mye*, and the Germans as, *vergiz min niht*. A German painting has a portrait of a young man on one side, the reverse shows a woman making a chaplet of forget-me nots, with the words, 'I bind with forget-me-nots.'

Wallflowers, *Erysimum cheiri*, are likely to have been brought to Britain as seed by the Normans when they began transporting stone from France to build their mighty castles and abbeys, where you may see wallflowers still growing on the ruined walls today. Wallflowers were one of the several gillyflowers, all of which were scented, the main ones being the clove gillyflowers, which are the pinks and carnations, and the stock gillyflowers, the highly scented stocks. Today, a person who is described as a wallflower is usually shy and retiring, but in medieval times, a wallflower would be worn to shown faithfulness to one lover only. A story tells how a young girl fell in love with a man who her father thought was unsuitable; he wanted her to marry the son of a local lord to forge a strong alliance. The girl and her beloved planned to elope. On the agreed night, she knotted sheets together, tied them to her bed and began to lower herself out of her window; but the sheets tore apart. She fell to her death. The grieving man plucked a wallflower from the castle wall as a memento and to show that he would remain loyal to her memory and love forever.

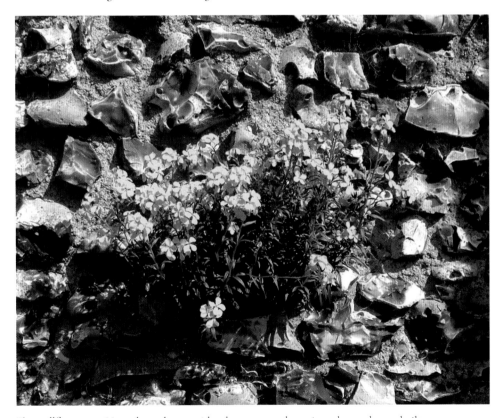

The wallflowers on Newark castle are said to have grown there since the castle was built.

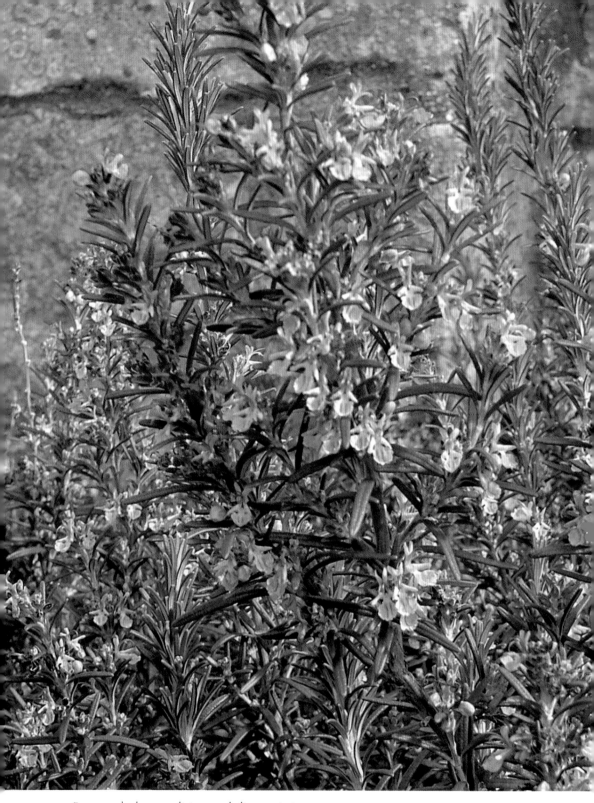

Rosemary had many religious symbolic associations.

Although many plants were named after the Virgin Mary, rosemary isn't one of them. The name means rose of the sea, as the plant grew on coastal areas of the Mediterranean. Rosemary may have been introduced into Britain by the Romans, but if it had been, it had disappeared or was rare by the medieval period. Rosemary must have been quite a novelty because Henry Daniel translated a short treatise on the culture of rosemary from a Latin text, originally from Salerno, which stated that the original document and some rosemary had been sent to England in 1338 by the Countess of Hainault to her daughter, Queen Phillipa, as until that time, rosemary was little known of in England. Daniel noted that rosemary had many virtues and he mentions sixty five! The flowers, which may appear twice a year, were considered to be more valuable than the leaves. Cold north easterly and easterly winds were likely to kill the rosemary bushes, so care was needed to help the plant to survive harsh winters. Such were the difficulties of growing rosemary that Daniel said that it only thrived for those people who were rightful and just! He then went on to describe how rosemary could be propagated by cuttings.

Mention is made of a belief that in suitable conditions, rosemary never grew taller than Christ when he had walked on the earth, although no measurement is given, and if a rosemary bush lived for more than thirty-three years, it would grow no higher, only broader. This comes from a medieval tradition that Christ died when he was thirty-three, making this the perfect age to be alive. The life and death of Christ had had its own plant symbolism. The elder was the tree from which Judas hanged himself. How he found an elder tree that was tall and strong enough is a miracle in itself. In European mythology, the elder would continue to have a bad reputation; the wood has few practical uses, nor does it burn well enough to make a good firewood, and it was reputed to be favoured by witches.

Easter was a major festival throughout Europe. To celebrate Palm Sunday most people were forced to improvise and use willow or yew branches, which were more easily found than real palm leaves. Some legends suggested that the crown of thorns was originally a rose briar, but there were more than enough other thorny plants that could be used to symbolise it. Louis IX of France acquired the crown of thorns as a result of the sacking of Constantinople in 1204 during the fourth Crusade. He later built the largest ever reliquary, St Chapelle, to house the crown in appropriate splendour. Constantinople was in possession of the True Cross, which it claimed had been found by the empress Helena. The Bible makes no mention of which wood the cross was made of, but by medieval times there were many stories of the cross that had been written to incorporate biblical references and to imply a continuity from the Old Testament into the New Testament; the cross being fashioned from the Tree of Knowledge of Good and Evil from the Garden of Eden. The Eastern Orthodox Church has a tradition that the cross was constructed of three different woods, cedar, cypress and pine. Strabo wrote that the bitter juice of wormwood represented the gall

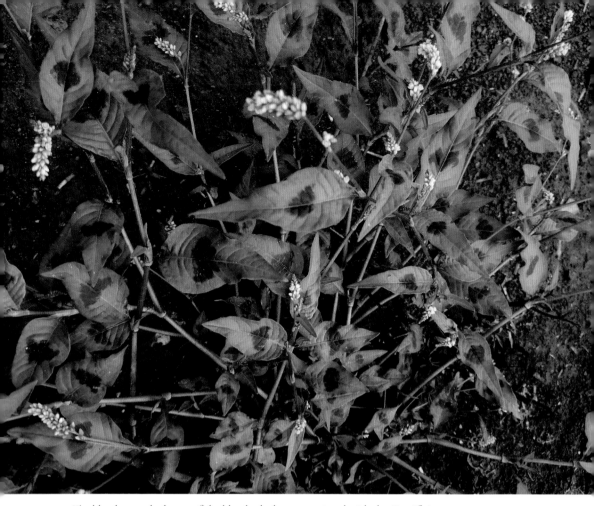

The blotches on the leaves of the bloody dock are associated with the Crucifixion.

offered to Christ during the crucifixion. Several plants acquired association with the crucifixion because their leaves were said to have been splattered with the blood of Christ as he hung on the cross, such as the bloody dock and the spotted orchid. The Cuckoo Pint often has green leaves but sometimes the leaves have purple spots.

Primroses have long been known as a harbinger of spring and all parts of the plant are edible, making them a useful food plant early in the year. The medieval English song, *Maid in the Moor Lay*, tells of a maiden who slept out on a moor for a week and a day. She was sustained by primroses and violet flowers with cold spring water as her drink. Protection from the cold was provided by a bower of red roses and lilies. All of the flowers are associated with the Virgin Mary, but the song may be about a humble maiden lost on a moor.

Many plants that we consider to be weeds are simply those plants for which we no longer have a use, and some of them have common names that date from medieval times. Shepherd's purse gets its name from the shape of the seed cases which resemble a medieval shepherd's purse; so much so that the name was contemporary even in the

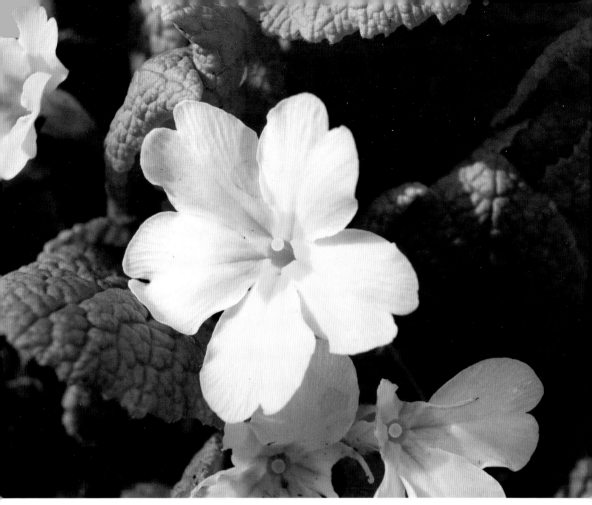

The primrose heralded the arrival of spring.

medieval period. If you hold the seed stalk at the bottom, the seedcase is similar to the medieval purses shown in illustrations. There are only two seeds, which represent the money in the purse, because shepherds were not wealthy! The main use of the plant was to staunch blood flow. As it is a common weed in fields and gardens, and can be found during most of the year, it was easily found if you were suffering from a bad cut when working in the fields. It also has a medieval name of toothwort to cure toothache, probably because the seedcases also appear vaguely like a tooth.

Along with docks and nettles, thistles were considered to be thuggish enough to be removed from crops, although they too had their uses. The young shoots of thistles were eaten to cleanse the system after spring purges that were common after the poor diet of winter. Herb bennet, *Geum urbanum*, is a common weed that most people today would readily remove, but according to one writer, we would be wrong to treat it so lightly. It was highly prized because, 'where the root is in the house, the Devil can do nothing and flies from it!'

CHAPTER 7

Magical and Mysterious

In medieval times the world existed in a web of unseen influences, for both good and evil. Plants were not exempt. Some plants are poisonous and have been used to destroy life. The same poisonous plant could be a beneficial medicinal plant, being used to put a patient to sleep so that the surgeon can cut them or possibly to carry out painful manoeuvres such as resetting a broken limb. Although the mandrake, *Mandragora officinarum*, would have been as rare in medieval Britain as it is today, people would have known of it, especially the tales about how dangerous it was to harvest the roots. The mandrake would scream when wrenched from the soil. If you heard the scream, you would surely die! If you were very lucky, you may only go mad! A knowledgeable person would be forewarned and well prepared.

Some instructions were complicated. In his encyclopaedia of nature, Bartholomew the Englishman warned that if you were going to dig up mandrake you should wait until sunset and beware of contrary winds. To ensure magical protection, the person who wished to dig up the root should draw three circles around the plant with a sword. Swords were expensive. It was much cheaper and less trouble to delicately loosen the roots of the mandrake plant, then tie a hungry hound to the plant. The person should retire to a safe distance, block their ears with wax as an extra precaution, then tempt the hound with a bowl of food. The hungry animal ran towards food, pulling the mandrake out of the ground, where upon it screamed, the dog died, and the plant collector survived another day. If you were wealthy enough to possess a sword, you could draw magical circles to protect yourself, but dogs were in plentiful supply.

The stories ensured that the roots sold at a good price, but it also scared off the less experienced collectors, so that young plants would be left alone to grow to maturity. The ripe fruits, known as apples of mandrake, were much easier to collect and there was no risk involved. Simply inhaling the scent of the fruit would send you to sleep, so it was said. People yearn for the mysterious, so there were many potential customers for mandrake roots. Most people would never see a real mandrake root, which meant that a trade in fake mandrakes was easy to carry out and profitable. White bryony is a common hedgerow plant that quickly produces a large, thick root. The root is like a mandrake root without any extra work, but with some careful carving, you

MEDIEVAL PLANTS AND THEIR USES

est iouis barba uncia una· rape semen uncia una· flar
tos titios uncia una· eupatorii uncia una· peto radicem
hec est capsella uncia una· erpeti uncia una· trifoli se
men quod mulieres in capite utuntur uncia una· a
moru uncia una· serpuli sicci uncia una· Centaure
uncia una· aristologie uncia una· rure agrestis untia
una· crute semen uncia una· Lacturadicem hec est si
psana siue armonia semen uncia una· puna semen un
cia una· hec omnia contunduntur in uno in puluere
lenissimu et ita cum melle attico teres bene commi
sces et sic condi ligent abis priburi decorne utere quo
moto uolueris· uel ante lucem dabis in magnitudine
abellane hec si usus fueris usq ad diem desinitionis
tue saluus eris.

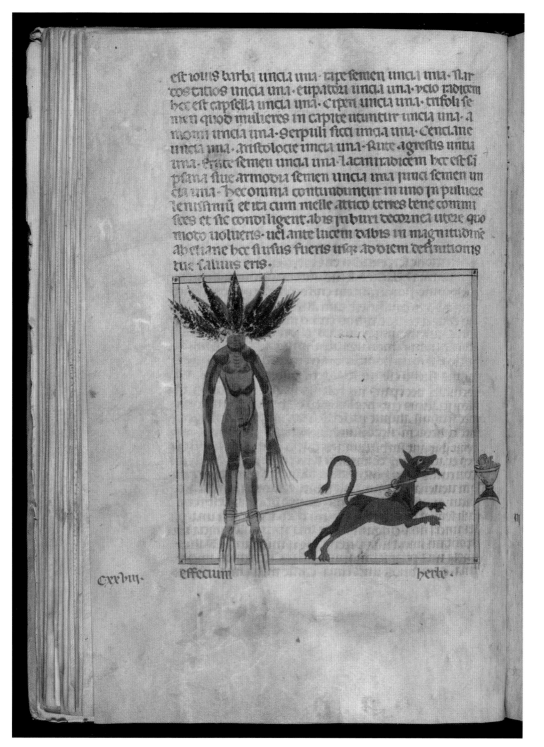

cxx·lviij·   effectum   herb·

Harvesting the mandrake root was a dangerous operation. (The Wellcome Collection)

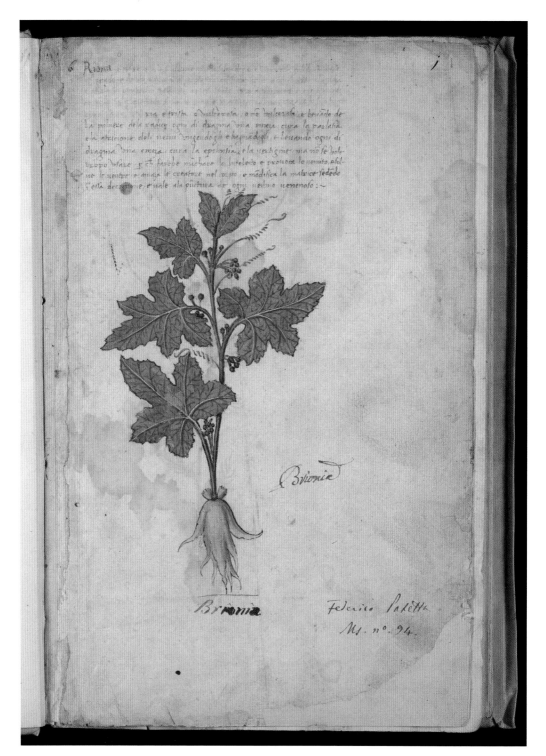

The root of white bryony has a similar appearance to that of the mandrake. (The Wellcome Collection)

could produce a root that had the appearance that most people expected of a real mandrake; and then sell the fake at a very handsome profit.

Cinnamon was another plant that attracted tales. It was said to be found in birds' nests, and especially the nest of the phoenix. Ash trees were such a magical plant that snakes would not go over a shadow cast by an ash tree. Snakes were so scared of the tree that if you placed a snake within a circle of ash leaves next to a fire, the snake would sooner throw itself into the flames than cross the circle of ash leaves. The shade of a yew tree was equally dangerous, as any person or beast that slept under a yew was certain to die.

Although Shakespeare was writing later, in his play *Macbeth*, the witches dig up hemlock roots in the dark of night, which is very practical advice if you want to avoid being seen harvesting poisonous plants by inquisitive and suspicious neighbours.

The marigold, *Calendula*, was thought to be a plant ruled by the sun as the flowers turn to face the sun throughout the day. The bright sunlight illuminates hidden things that are in darkness, so placing marigold flowers under your pillow at night would reveal in a dream the whereabouts of anything that had been lost or stolen and the person who was the thief. A person who picked a marigold flower in August, the month of Leo and the sun, and wrapped it in a bay leaf with a wolf's tooth would ensure that nobody could speak ill of them for as long as they carried the package.

Vervain, *Verbena officinalis*, is a plant that most people today would scarcely notice. The plant does not grow very tall, it has spindly stems, small leaves and tiny white

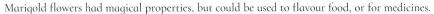

Marigold flowers had magical properties, but could be used to flavour food, or for medicines.

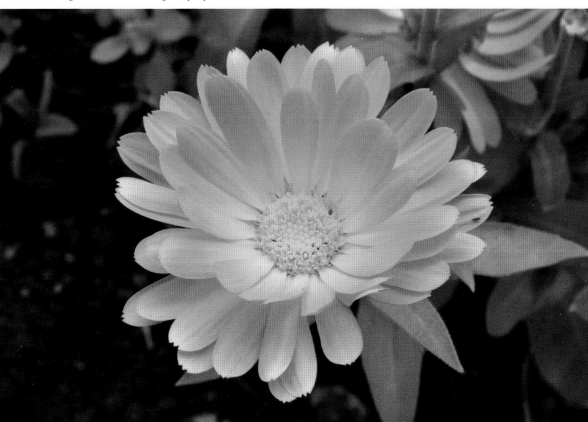

flowers. It is easy to pass it by, yet for some reason, it has a mass of folklore and a magical reputation attached to it. This was mostly because of the writings of Pliny who was copied for centuries to come with little contradiction. He named the plant as a holy herb, but which plant he was writing about is uncertain. Later medieval writers believed that he meant *Verbena officinalis*. Pliny gave many medicinal uses for the vervain, but some were more magical than medicinal; for example, you could bind a piece of vervain to an aching head, and this would cure all headaches, whatever their cause. Pliny also said that witches praised vervain because it could cure all ills, but for later writers, it could do much more. Crush the plant and rub the juice over your body, and any wish that you make will be granted! Putting it in your house or growing it on your land or in your vineyard was an assured way to give you increased profits and an abundance of revenue. The *Macer Herbal* claimed that a man who held a sprig of vervain in his hand would not be barked at by dogs, regardless of his intent. Then, after giving many different medical cures that made use of vervain, towards the end of the chapter we are given the cautionary warning. 'Other such many, they say the which, through peradventure the mighty nature may grant, that it seems thus that they be not but idle sayings'!

To be forever merry, which you may think really does require magic, you only had to add saffron to your food and drink, so you would need the aforementioned abundance of revenue to be able to afford the cost of saffron! Following this regime, you would never be sad again, but you did have to be careful; if you ate too much saffron, you risked dying of an excess of joy!

Vervain has many small flowers that are similar to stars from a distance.

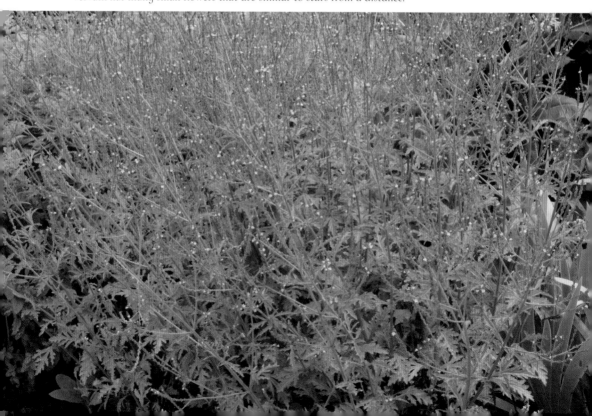

Peony was a prized plant in the medieval garden. There were two types, the male peony, *Paeonia mascula*, which has pale cerise petals and the female peony, *Paeonia officinalis*, with red flowers. During the medieval period both would have had open flowers with single petals, not the multi-petal forms that are mostly grown in gardens today. As with many other plants, peony had medical virtues, but some of them were magical too. The *Macer Herbal* repeated the story first told by Galen of how to cure children suffering from the falling sickness, which is probably epilepsy. Galen recounted that once upon a time he saw a child of about eight years old who did indeed have the falling evil. To counteract the malady, the child had be given a peony root on a cord to wear around his neck, which kept him safe. Somehow, the root fell from the child's neck, and he soon fell to the earth. The root was quickly tied around his neck, and soon the child was well again! Galen marvelled at this, so he experimented by removing the

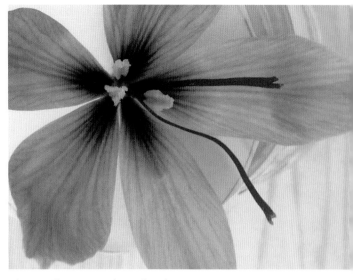

Above: Saffron was said to induce happiness.

Below: The flowers of the male peony are much paler than those of the female peony.

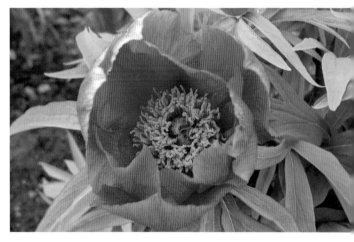

root, and sure enough, the child fell to the ground. When Galen replaced the root around the child's neck, he was healed. And this was how Galen said that he learned for certain the virtue of the peony. His ideas would be repeated for centuries to come.

To be able to grasp hot metal or resist being burned by flames you should mix the juice of hollyhocks, psyllium seeds, *Plantago ovata*, with those of the fleabane, *Pulicaria dysenterica*, and the juice of radish. Pulverise them all together and mix into the white of an egg. Wash the liquid onto your hand, allow it to dry and repeat the process once more, again allowing the liquid to dry on your skin. You can now grasp red hot metal with no ill effect. Believe it if you will!

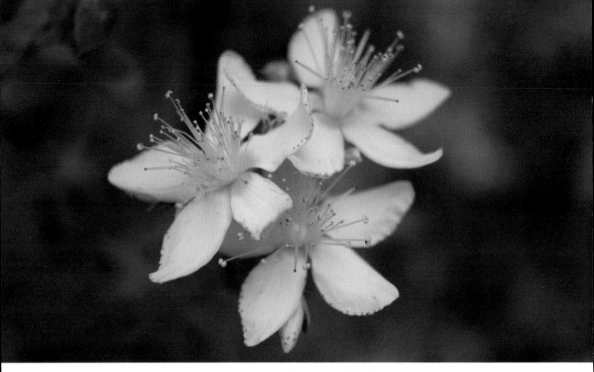

Saint John's wort expelled demons and was made into an oil for skin complaints.

Possession by devils was well-known to most people through bible stories. The demons may visit you in your dreams, so to sleep without such dreams, you could hang vervain around your neck and drink some of the juice before going to bed. If you had been possessed by spirits, Saint John's wort was one of the main plants that could be drunk as a medicine to drive them out of your body. More recent research has shown that the herb is useful for treating depression, the symptoms of which can be much the same as being possessed by evil spirits!

Another remedy suitable for those possessed by evil spirits or for mad men was to wrap an 'affodill' bulb in clean linen and carry it on their person, although it is unclear whether the plant intended was the daffodil or the asphodel. Some people believed that the devil and evil spirits would be deterred by ferns. Anybody who carried fern about their body as protection would not suffer from apparitions nor the ill effects of demonic curses or magical spells. Another benefit of carrying ferns was that if you had been poisoned, the poison would become ineffective.

Simply holding nettle and yarrow stems in your hand would free you from fear, visions and fantasies, whilst keeping the herb mugwort in your house would ensure that no ghosts or evil spirits would be able to live there. Some cures were specific to a set time. To be cured of the madness that was caused by evil spirits, you must go out on mid-summer's night, between midnight and the dawn, and collect the best green walnut leaves that you can find. The leaves should be distilled in water on the same day, after sunrise, but before sunset. Drink the water and you would be cured of the madness. One herbal was not bothered about the medical uses of Saint John's wort but was keen to point out that if the plant was kept in a house, then no wicked ghosts could either enter, or remain there if they had already taken up residence. The smoke of birthwort could be used to drive away all devils, with the bonus that it would bring cheer to young children. Wearing betony about your person would deter even the Devil, although the church preferred that it was the only authority that should be consulted on matters of possession by demons or evil spirits. At an official exorcism, the officiating priest would sprinkle holy water using the branches of rue to drive away the evil spirits. Bunches of herbs such as hyssop and rosemary were used to sprinkle holy water on other occasions. To get the better of all your enemies, you should carry some greater celandine and the heart of a mole. This would allow you to win all your causes and triumph in debates.

With many houses being thatched, the risk of house fires was high, so any assistance to avoid the thunder bolts of Zeus was welcome. This led the emperor Charlemagne to decree that his subjects should grow houseleeks on their roofs so that they would not be struck by lightning. This was easy to achieve as houseleeks grow happily on walls and roofs with little soil, which in itself, may once have appeared to be magical for many people. Fires in thatch roofs were common, so if you were burned or scalded trying to put out the fire, the leaves of the houseleeks could be applied to the injured part to bring relief.

A successful harvest was a constant worry to most farmers as it would ensure that you would not starve before the following one. Hailstorms could quickly flatten a grain crop which would have grown much taller than modern crops, which may cause the crop to rot before the harvest. It was thought that if ferns were grown in the fields, then hail would rarely fall on them, nor would lightning strike them.

Houseleeks could be grown on the roof to avoid being struck by lightning.

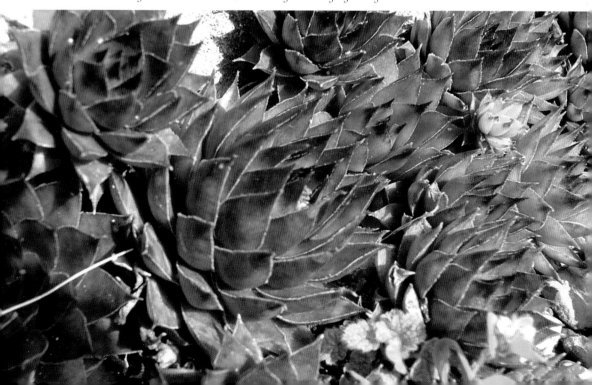

CHAPTER 8

Love, Seduction and Beauty

Making yourself attractive to the opposite sex and seducing a lover often relied on plants, many of which are best not attempted today. Presenting an enticing image to the potential lover was all, but it required care. For Christian women there was a fine line between looking their best and arousing criticism from the church, which with good reason suspected that any improvement on God-given beauty would lead to sinful lusting. The crusades had been responsible for exposing western Europeans to exotic perfumes and new cosmetic methods, whilst the art of distillation, perfected by the Arabs, had enabled them to produce alcohol based perfumes, which were preferable to the ones that had been available previously which were based on oil or fat.

During the medieval period, there were many cosmetics available, if you could afford them. For those with little money, word-of-mouth may have passed on traditional methods that were not recorded. Many herbals included cosmetics and beauty tips. There was one writer who was believed to have spoken from the experience of being a woman. Trota of Salerno, sometimes known as Dame Trot may have been the wife of a physician, although this is not certain, and some modern historians still doubt whether the author of the works was actually a woman.

Works have been genuinely attributed to Trota, whether as a female or a male author. A compilation of Trota's writings and those of other authors became known as the, *Trotula*.

A picture of a female physician, who may represent Dame Trotula. (The Wellcome Collection)

Trotula was later mistakenly believed to be the name of the female author of the whole compilation, rather than the book itself. The later *Trotula* included recipes for cosmetics, conception, contraception, and childbirth. First, you had to attract your man. Cosmetics could be used to enhance a woman's beauty.

Skin Preparations

Lilies and roses appear in many poetic descriptions of medieval high-born ladies. A medieval maid of high birth was usually described in comparison to the two most-loved flowers. Her pale face was to be the pure white colour of the Madonna lily, whilst her cheeks were to be blushed with the pink of roses. This was the ideal for the ladies of the elite classes who had the leisure time and the money to achieve it. During his quest to find the Green Knight, Gawain finds himself alone in bed, at risk of seduction by his host's Sir Bertilak's beautiful wife, who he notices is:

> *Wyth chynne and cheke ful swete,*
> *Bothe quit and red in blande,*
> *Ful lufly con ho lete,*
> *Wyth lyppes smal laghande.*

A lady of high birth would have a smooth, unblemished pale or white skin to show off her status. She was certainly not getting her pale complexion ruined by the sun and wind as a result of having to work in the fields! The paleness was exaggerated with cosmetics to give a distinctly white colour. The Virgin Mary was supposed to be a carpenter's wife, yet as the Queen of Heaven, her face was mostly depicted as being white, the same as the other ladies of high birth. Other than keeping out of the sun, there were ways to enhance your skin tone and to enhance the whiteness. Some women were prepared go to great lengths to achieve the ideal.

For the lady who wanted a white, clear face or generally to remove blemishes and make the skin paler, there were many plants that could be used. She could make an ointment of fresh pork fat, the white of an egg and mix them together with powdered bay leaves. She could make a mix of the root of bistort crushed with cuttlefish and frankincense. Not all the plant-based recipes were particularly risk free. The wild arum, often known as lords and ladies, and its larger relative, the medieval dragon plant, both have roots that contain an alkaloid that can cause serious blistering of the skin. This is not a recipe to try at home:

> Take the roots of either Dragons or Lords and Ladies and place them in a
> container of rose water and leave the container in the sun until the water has

been absorbed. Dry the roots, then crush them into a powder. Rub the powder on your face, or whatever place you wish to be fair, two or three times, and then wash your skin where you had placed the powder with rose water, and you shall be fair. The powder also takes away surplus flesh where a person is troubled by rough or coarse skin on the face and it will become much cleaner and more lovely than using white lead.

With the modern footnote, that it would be safer in the long term than using the lead-based ceruse as a method of making the skin whiter.

Another common plant still grown in gardens today is the caper spurge. Do not be tempted to eat the seeds in the belief that they are capers. The name, spurge, tells you that this is a purging plant! The caper spurge is a member of the euphorbia family, most of which have caustic saps that can cause blistering of the skin, so it was ideal as a cosmetic to make the face whiter. To use the caper spurge safely, it was thoroughly crushed and cooked in honey and then mixed with an equal quantity of wine.

Welks, which we know as acne, is a problem that still causes embarrassment, but could be simply resolved with an ointment made by pounding the roots of docks, then frying them in grease. Spots and freckles have always been a problem for some people, although others find freckles attractive. A plaster of celandine leaves ground with wine was used to destroy and wipe away spots and freckles. The juice of the stinking iris could be used to remove wrinkles by rubbing the juice onto the wrinkled skin in

Caper spurge could be used to make the face a paler colour.

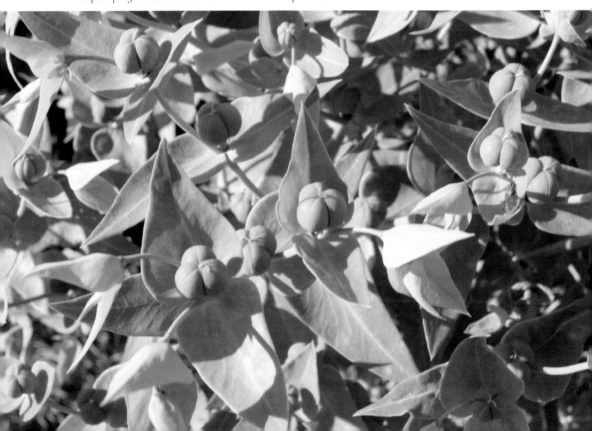

the evening before bed. In the morning rub off the blistered skin to leave a delicate skin. The juice of wild celery washed on the face would have the same effect. Simply drinking chamomile tea was said to remove spots or freckles.

TO REMOVE FRECKLES

Take the roots of the wild iris. Make them into a powder, and add vinegar and dry them, and temper it with rose water and dry it. Do this for three or four times more. Rub with this powder and rose water and in doing this, remove the freckles and clean them from your face.

If you cut yourself, mix catmint with oil of roses to clear any wound and prevent the unsightly marks of a scar. The oil would also refresh the bloom of the skin and was even said to restore hair. Some women may have wished to make their faces appear to have more redness in the cheeks. A cosmetic rouge could be produced in several ways. Wash the roots of red and white bryony then cut in small pieces and dry them. Next, crush the pieces to make a fine powder and mix in a quantity of rose water. With a fine cloth of linen or cotton, wash the face with the liquid, which will cause the skin to turn red. Bryony roots can cause inflammation, so the recipe probably would be effective although if the mixture was too powerful you may have blistering of the face. A safer method would be to use pieces of the imported tree wood, brazilwood, as a dye to give a good pinkish colour that could be applied as a concentrated liquid. Another recipe suggested that the lady mix the root of the iris in a large quantity of bear's grease and the root of marshmallow and put them in wine and oil for ten days and then simmer the mix and add to it the colour that is put in sealing wax and some oil and use the ointment to colour the face.

Cosmetics would be available to buy from the local apothecary, for those who could afford them. There were other more unlikely sources too. The Italian painter, Cennino d'Andrrea Cennini, wrote in his book about artistic methods, *Il Libro dell' Arte*, that ladies would buy colours from artists to use as cosmetics. He did not approve, giving the usual opinion that it was not the will of God, nor that of the Virgin Mary, for women to enhance their beauty with cosmetics. He then wrote that if a woman wished to remain beautiful, she should wash using pure water from a spring, river or well. For the ladies who did use cosmetics, there were perils, he warned; these women risked their complexion becoming withered and their teeth would be turned black. They would soon appear to be older than they actually were 'like the most hideous women that you could imagine'. And with that brief tirade, he finished his discussion on the matter of cosmetics.

Veins on the face were to be removed by mixing three parts of soap to one part of pepper, powder the mix and wash the skin with it. A lady should have soft, smooth skin, without any body hair. Removing unwanted body hair is easily carried out with wax or electronics today, but one medieval recipe promised to remove unwanted hair for ever. A depilatory ointment to remove body hair could be made using the juice of squirting cucumber (not readily available in Britain) and almond milk placed in a vessel with quicklime and orpiment. Add powdered galbanum with some wine. Quicklime alone would certainly do the job, without any other ingredients.

The medieval ideal was generally for the woman to have small lips highlighted with a red salve similar to a modern lipstick. A red-stained beeswax ointment produces a good effect; although my own experiments gave a good colour, it came off the lips very quickly and needed frequent replacement. A woman's crowning glory was often her hair, but there were restrictions on how you were allowed to display your hair. A young unmarried woman could flaunt long flowing hair, but a married woman or a nun was expected to hide her hair so that she would not unwittingly arouse the attention of male admirers. Blonde hair was as desirable during the medieval period as it is now, but disguising grey hair was thought to be nothing more than vanity; but that was not going to stop people trying. The commonest bleach to lighten hair colour was the lye which was applied to the hair and left to soak. Lye was produced by pouring fresh water through the ashes of burned hardwoods., Lye is caustic, so needed handling with care. If you get lye on your fingers, your skin will have a soapy feel to it. This is your skin dissolving! If you experiment with lye, handle it with great care. The green, outer skin of the walnut produces a dark brown dye that could be used to dye hair. I knew somebody who used to dye her hair with onion skins. Another recipe to make a dark hair colourant is given in the *Trotula*. Burn oak apples in oil and then pulverise them before adding vinegar and a blackening mix used by shoemakers. Oak apples were used to make a black ink, so this would certainly work.

Ladies were expected to have a high forehead, forcing them to pluck or shave the hairs at the front of the head. Eyebrows were plucked to produce a high arch form, with charcoal or lamp black applied to enhance them where suitable. Young women were allowed to show off their hair and could spend some time perfecting its appearance. One of the easiest ways to keep hair looking its best was by regular brushing to keep it tangle-free and shiny. To perfume your hair, you could make a powder of dried rose petals, cloves, nutmeg, watercress, and galangal, then stir in some water. Dip your comb into the liquid before combing your hair to make it smell sweeter. Musk or cloves were other substances for scenting hair. Dandruff is unsightly but thankfully, *Trotula* gave a recipe to help to get rid of it. Collect nettle seeds and soak them for two to three days in vinegar. Wash your hair with a good soap, then soak your hair with the vinegar. Cider vinegar is still used by many people as a hair wash to rebalance the pH of the scalp after using a shampoo and nettles are still included in some modern shampoos. Soap was produced using a mixture of fats and

MEDIEVAL PLANTS AND THEIR USES

wood lye. Having made the soap, it must be left to stand for a few months to allow the pH to become less caustic. The most sought after soap was that known as Castile soap, which was made with olive oil. It was very expensive, making it a luxury item. Soapwort is a rapidly spreading plant, sometimes known as bouncing Bet, as it tends to fall over rather than standing upright. The leaves, stems and roots contain a 'soap' that can be used to wash the hair. Take several handfuls of the stems and leaves. Tear them into pieces and leave to soak in water overnight. Bring the water to the boil then simmer. Strain the water to remove the plant material and use the water to wash your hair. Unlike modern shampoos, you will not have bubbles, but your hair will be cleansed. If you stir the liquid vigorously, bubbles will form, but they will soon disappear.

The main problems with hair, especially for men, are to stop it falling out or encouraging it to grow from bald patches and to colour any grey hairs. To make hair grow again you could boil willow leaves in oil and lay the pulp where you want the hair to grow.

Scald head is a name given to the condition where there are pustules that form dried, scaly scurf on the head, often with the hair falling out. The herbalist Bernard Gordon provided a recipe:

> Take half an ounce each of- litharge, sulphur, wine, chalk, bibbey (An unknown ingredient), arenment, vitriol, orpiment, soot, verdigris, hellebores white and black, alum and galls. Half a pound of each of wax, pitch, oil of almonds. Then the juice of mallows, fumitory, scabious, borage, a quarter of a pound. Boil the oil, wax and pitch with the juices until the juices have gone, then add the other ingredients to complete the ointment.

Fumitory is a wildflower that is easily overlooked. It gets its name because if there are lots of plants growing close together, they do resemble a cloud of smoke when seen from a distance.

The roots of affadilla could be burned to a powder and the ashes rubbed into the scalp where the hair has been lost would make the hair grow again. Burn southernwood and mix the ashes with old oil, then apply to the place that lacks hair, and hey presto! The hair shall be restored again. You could try boiling willow leaves in oil and laying the mush where you want the hair to grow, or slightly smellier, you could grind red onions into a paste and rub that on the bald areas. To help more serious hair loss, such as alopecia, simmer fresh scabious and teasels together, strain the water and wash it on the scalp.

A useful cosmetic was made by mixing catmint with oil of roses as an ointment, which was alleged to heal cuts, remove scars, restore the freshness of the skin and restore hair loss caused by a septic cut.

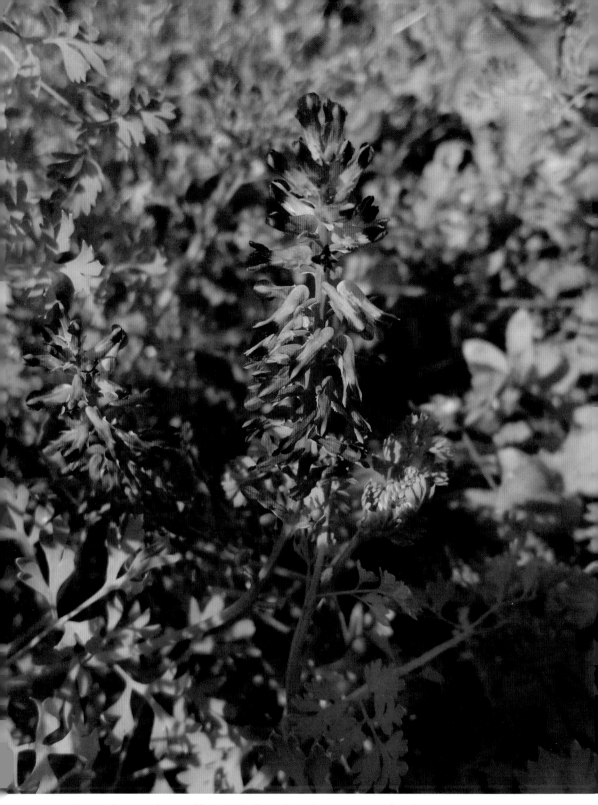

From a distance, clumps of fumitory in flower have the appearance of smoke.

MEDIEVAL PLANTS AND THEIR USES

Nits could be killed by washing your hair with water that had been left to stand with white bryony root, which is a much safer option than the mercury, orpiment or quicklime that some recipes suggested.

Having improved the complexion, most women know that the hands can ruin the whole scheme. Hands could be made whiter by boiling wild garlic leaves in water until it has evaporated. Mix in two eggs and tartar and wash your hands. Clean, attractive fingernails were not a fashion option for somebody who was working in the fields or using dyes or other industrial processes that caused stains. A lady, on the other hand, could keep her nails clean and unbroken very easily. If you had bad finger or toenails you could tie the berries of danewort, sometimes known as dwarf elder, to the nails. The bad nails would fall off and beautiful new nails would grow in their place.

If all had gone to plan, but too many kisses the night before had caused your lips to crack, rub them with an ointment containing lilies or fleabane. For sore lips, thoroughly crush the roots of knapweed mixed with cow's cream, and then strained through a clean piece of cloth. Dab the liquid on your lips to ease the soreness. Oil of roses or violets with some wax melted in it would make an excellent lip balm. Another lip cream could be used for sunburn too. Boil lily bulbs in water, then drain and crush the bulbs. Add melted pork fat. Stir in an ounce each of powdered mastic, frankincense, and two scruples each of white lead and camphor and some rose water. In the evening you should sit by the fire to let your face warm before applying the ointment. It would not need to be washed off in the morning either.

A lady was expected to have eyes that were clear and shining. There is a late medieval reference to Italian ladies using the juice of deadly nightshade in their eyes to make their pupils dilate, which helps to make a woman more attractive to men; the plant's common name, belladonna, means beautiful lady. Atropine derived from the plant is still used by doctors to open the pupil. You experience a sudden increase of light and then blurred vision for an hour or more. Another theory is that the bella comes from the Latin word for war, as deadly nightshade is a good painkiller and sedative if used correctly.

If you suffered from very bad body odour, rose oil would cover some offensive smells, but it was a very expensive luxury item for a good reason. Today it takes 5000kg/833lbs of *Rosa Gallica* petals per hectare, to produce only one kilo of oil. Rose oil is one of the main ingredients in Chanel No 5. A cheaper alternative was Hungary Water, which some claim was the first European perfume that was alcohol-based. It is thought to have been invented during the mid-fourteenth century. Legend tells that the Queen Elizabeth of Hungary, aged seventy-two, was suffering from gout and other ills that were brought on by her old age. An elderly hermit is said to have given her the recipe, before disappearing; never to be seen again. The water was so powerful, that the queen regained her youthful appearance and received an offer of marriage from the king of Poland, which she refused. Most of the legends seem to date from centuries later and may have been added by apothecaries to lend an air of mystery to their product to attract more customers! The distilled water was to be both drunk and applied to the body. The main ingredients were the tops and flowers of rosemary distilled in aqua vitae. A simple replica could be made by soaking the rosemary leaves in vodka. A similar elixir was Carmelite Water, reputed to have been first produced by the Carmelite nuns of the Abbey Saint Juste during the fourteenth century. The alcohol-based distillation's main ingredient is balm, often called lemon balm, *Melissa officinalis*, but other plant ingredients can be used. The water could be drunk or applied to the body.

Those with less money could boil bilberry leaves or the berries themselves in wine and wash themselves with the liquid. A bath of water with lovage leaves helped to give the body a wholesome odour and acted as a deodorant.

The perfect teeth were to be white, the idea of high-status people having black teeth as a result of eating lots of expensive sugar would not become fashionable until the Elizabethan times. Teeth were cleaned with toothpicks. Toothpicks made of wood, or a feather quill may have been used. Silver or copper alloy utensils have been found across most of Europe that have an ear scoop at one end and a point at the other, which may be a toothpick or could have been used to clean the fingernails. The use of toothbrushes in the west is generally said to date from the late eighteenth century, although there is a medieval French reference to them. A simple toothbrush brush can be made by

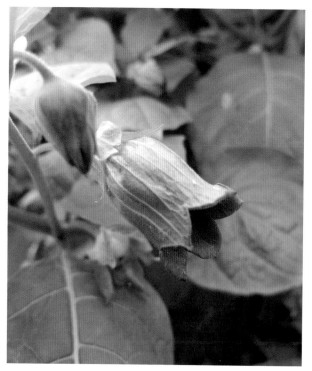

hammering the end of a stick to separate the fibres. Sage leaves are coarse and can be rubbed on the teeth to clean them, with the bonus of freshening the breath. Whether this was a method used by medieval people is uncertain, but one recipe for cleaning the teeth says that you should crush sage leaves with a mortar and add an equal amount of salt. Make the mix into small pastilles then place them in a hot oven until they are black and burned. The powder can

Deadly nightshade could be used as a cosmetic or a painkiller.

MEDIEVAL PLANTS AND THEIR USES

be used to rub on the teeth that are yellow, rotten or stinking. Poor dental hygiene would encourage bad breath and not make you attractive to the opposite sex. Chewing fresh fennel seeds would sweeten the breath as would mint leaves. Mouthwashes could be made by simmering mint leaves in water or wine or dissolving myrrh into wine. If bad breath was caused by a stomach disorder, crush the tips of myrtle in wine and simmer to reduce by half. Drink after purging. Another remedy for bad breath was to take the juice of orpine, *Sedum telephium*, feverfew, angelica, and pennyroyal. Mix them with some honey. Take a spoonful at night and morning. Rosemary leaves and flowers simmered in white wine with a small amount of myrrh and pellitory on the wall would give wonderful results if you gargled with it regularly.

MEDIEVAL TOOTHPASTES

To clean black teeth or those that were not very white, rub the teeth with a clean walnut shell three times a day, followed by washing the mouth with warm wine to which salt can be added if you wish. A more refined toothpaste was made by mixing cinnamon, cloves, spikenard, frankincense, mastic, grain, date and olive stones and a crab's foot and grinding them to a powder. This would also sweeten the breath. Another paste could be made of equal parts of salt and pumice stone. Heat them over a fire in a plain dish until they burn. Grind them to a powder, adding a small amount of cinnamon and cloves to flavour it. The juice of scarlet pimpernel not only whitened teeth it was a cure for inflammation of the gums.

Love Potions and Aphrodisiacs

Sexual desire is often encountered in medieval herbals for one of two reasons, to help produce children or as an underhand method to encourage an uninterested partner. Inducing sexual desire as an aid to seduction is nothing new; it is usually an underhand method to encourage an uninterested partner without them being aware. Encouraging the feel-good-factor is a good start, so adding a nutmeg to food or drink was said to open the heart and make you feel joyful. Recent research has shown that larger quantities of nutmeg can induce a sense of euphoria, but in excess, this can lead to death. Perfume oils and waters can have a similar effect without any risks. Roses, lilies, violets and spices are still used in modern perfumery. One herbal suggested that the woman could dust a powder of bay leaves, cloves, galingale, nutmeg and dried rose petals on her breasts, nipples and genitals before sexual intercourse. Plying the person of your desire with alcohol may help, but with too much wine, things may not turn out as expected! Leek juice would prevent drunkenness, but how this could be administered is another matter.

Flatulence can be a laughing matter, but in certain social situations it can cause acute embarrassment, especially at a crucial moment during seduction; at such times a carminative, a remedy that expels flatulence or prevents it comes in handy. Avoiding foods that produce flatulence, such as beans and onions would be a good idea. Adding dill, fennel, mint, and savory to your food may help to prevent it.

If the person you are attempting to seduce resists you, a love potion or aphrodisiac could be used to entice the person you desired, or as an aid to make yourself appear more desirable to them. A medieval Dutch recipe claimed to be no less than the famous love potion that had been drunk by Tristan and Isolde in their story of ill-starred love. The aphrodisiac contained the petals of double red roses, so it was unlikely to lead to the same heights of passion portrayed in the story. Less safe was mandrake, which was known as an effective aphrodisiac and to be an aid to female fertility. Mandrake is toxic and would need to be used with care. For a man, wearing henbane about your person would ensure that women would fall in love with you. To improve sex drive or improve your performance, mallow was claimed to excite and prick lechery in either sex.

Vervain was another plant that gave strength for venereal pastimes and eating aniseed would increase the sex-drive in both men and women. Whereas you would think that women wanting to stir their own lust could find a better method than to eat raw onions!

Caraway provoked lechery but had the unfortunate side-effect of rapidly inducing urine. Drinking fennel seed mixed with wine sounds a much pleasanter way of stirring lechery.

There were even ways for a woman to deceive a man into believing that she had not lost her virginity. Most of the methods were intended to constrict the vagina. The treatise *De Curis Muliererum*, On the Treatment of Women, instructed that you should take the powdered mineral alum, (although later recipes mistake the words and use the whites of six eggs), and mix it with water in which hot herbs such as pennyroyal have been simmered. Soak a new, clean piece of linen in the liquid and insert it into the vagina two or three times a day. Alum is an astringent, so may produce the desired effect, egg whites would not. A similar method used the new-grown bark from a holm oak simmered with rainwater, which was applied in the same way, with a timely reminder not to forget to remove the linen.

Unwanted pregnancy before marriage was to be avoided. If this occurred it was assumed to be the woman's fault, a result of the Sin of Eve. The Bible suggests that Adam was a complete innocent until Eve was created to be his companion and was deceived by the serpent. The Church allowed sex, but only to produce offspring within wedlock. It was a necessary sin; it was to be endured solely to continue the human race. Pleasure was not meant to be an option. Despite evidence to the contrary, it was women who were thought to be the most likely to seek out sexual pleasure. In the case of an unwanted pregnancy, the poisonous plants were often used to induce an abortion. The herbals of the time mention this, but doctors were understandably wary of passing on the information to the general public. Most people could not read, and most herbals were mostly written in Latin, so this information was only accessible to a few people. The traditional use of plants used for contraception and abortion by the wider population is not recorded, but both may have been practised to limit the number of children who would need to be fed. This use of plants is still known and used in some parts of the world today, but the risks of permanent injury or death are very real.

Contraception was not a new idea. There were many medicines that could be taken to avoid or deal with pregnancy and many of the ideas were ancient. Plato had written that if too many children were being born, there were ways to control the population. The Greek physician Soranus of Ephesus wrote as early as the second century that a contraception would prevent the conception of a child, whereas an abortifacient removed that which had already been conceived. His own preference was for the safer contraception. The classical herbals recorded many plants to reduce human fertility. The most famous early contraceptive was a plant known as silphion or silphium, a species *ferula*, the giant fennel. It grew in one place only, the area around the Greek city-state of Cyrene in a mountainous strip of land along the eastern coast of Libya. It must have been a very potent drug as Soranus wrote that the woman only needed to swallow a

piece of the dried sap that was the size of a chickpea with water once a month for an effective method of birth control. Silphium had other uses as it was used in cookery and medicinally to treat coughs, stomach ailments, sore throats and fevers. The plant was of huge monetary value and was a major item for export, and for this reason, despite failed attempts to grow it elsewhere, the plant was harvested until there were no more plants in existence. The memory of Silphium survives only in the many written references and pictorial depictions on coins and carvings.

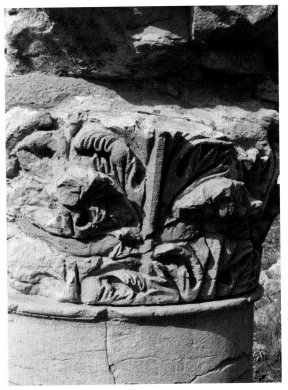

Silphium carved on a column at Cyrene, north-east Libya.

Luckily there were many other alternatives available. Pennyroyal, *Mentha pugelium*, was mentioned as a method of birth control by Aristophanes in his play, *Peace*, early in the fourth century BCE. Even today, herbalists know of the ability of pennyroyal to cause a miscarriage. The genus of plants called *Artemisia*, were named after the goddess Artemisia, who among her many other responsibilities, presided over women and childbirth. One of the more potent plants was wormwood, *Artemisia absinthium*, which was recorded by Dioscorides to be an anti-fertility drug and later gained the reputation of causing abortions. In more modern times it has also been proven to reduce sperm production. Rue, *Ruta graveolens*, was noted by Pliny the Elder to cause blisters if exposed skin was brushed against it in bright sunshine but is another toxic plant that could cause an abortion, with most modern herbals suggesting that it should not be eaten at all. Most modern herbals warn pregnant women not to eat juniper and its relative, savin, although the berries are often used in sauces for meats such as venison.

Most anti-fertility preparations were to be drunk by the woman, and many may have been completely ineffectual to prevent conception; mint juice applied to the vagina was said to ensure that a woman would not conceive at that time; yet recent research has shown that some plants do produce female sex hormones that to some measure, can prevent conception. Some of the plants may also affect male fertility by reducing the production of sperm. Most of the medicines were to be taken by the woman after intercourse in order to provoke the menses and a miscarriage. Some ingredients were poisonous and could prove fatal if the dosage was too strong. Oil of lilies was said to induce the menses by anointing the woman's body from the navel downwards. Another use was to bring relief to sore teats.

Savin had medicinal properties but was useful as an evergreen plant in gardens.

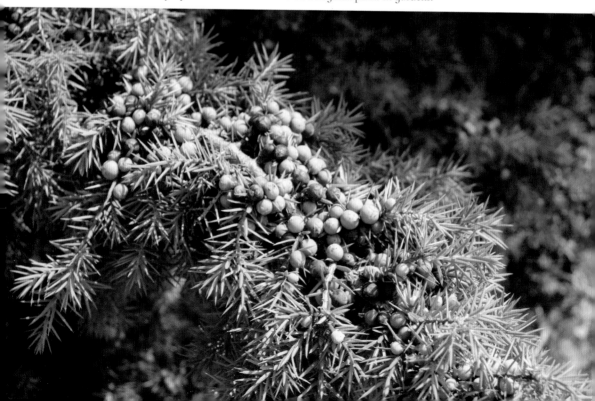

> ## OIL OF LILIES
> Take fresh lily flowers and put them in a container with olive oil. Leave to stand in the sun for nine days. Strain the oil through a cloth and leave to stand and settle for another nine days, then put into a glass bottle or a pot and seal the top. Other oils can be made using this method.

In modern times there is a clear distinction between contraception and induced, early abortions. This was not so clearly defined in the past. Hebrew Law, which influenced much of later Christian thinking, stated that a woman was not officially pregnant until forty days after conception. This left a prolonged period of leeway when an abortion was not technically unlawful. This argument has not gone away. There are many reasons that a woman may need to induce an early-stage abortion. Her own health may be at risk, or the foetus may be dead. Much of the formal information was recorded in herbals, but there must have been an oral-based tradition which has mostly been lost.

Male Sexual Problems

The penis was a symbol of manhood, so there were many ways to ensure that it looked its best. If it was swollen or sore, mash betony with a little wine, lay it on the penis and, 'It shall be healed!' And if a man lays the powder of dill seed on his penis, 'he shall be whole and no matter what manner of evil be on his penis, it shall heal it.' Impotence could be solved by soaking birch in water and drinking it.

Sexual performance has caused many men worries. With the absence of Viagra, there were many herbal remedies that would hopefully avoid embarrassment. The seed of rocket, especially the wild one, shall make the male member rise! Henbane came under the dominion of Jupiter, henbane seems to have been a powerful early form of Viagra, as it would allow a man to carry out the act of generation, very often! Henbane may work if taken internally, but it is poisonous. Be very careful not to get the dosage wrong...

The common knotgrass, *Polygonum aviculare*, was another medieval enhancer of potency, as drinking the juice would allow a man to perform coitus often! Fleabane eaten as a powder had a reputation to stir lust too, with the added bonus of removing intestinal worms.

Houseleeks could induce a man to such lusting that he would become, 'as if he was mad'. If houseleeks were cooked with milk and eggs and eaten for a few days, they would cure sterility in a man, but not a woman.

The Dragon plant is related to *Arum maculatum*, which today is often known as Wake Robin, which suggests knowledge of its use as a performance enhancer.

The juice of both plants has been rubbed onto the penis, but the juice is caustic, and whether drunk or applied, ought to arouse apprehension, as much as anything else!

Over-indulgence may cause its own problems. Swollen testicles were to be washed two or three times a day with a mixture of marshmallow, vervain, southernwood, henbane, mugwort and cabbages that had been simmered in old wine.

One writer claimed that 'Leeches say that this ointment will help swollen bollocks and other sores that affect the genitals, but it will work better if boiled beans are added to the mixture.'

Gilbertus the Englishman recommended that a man suffering from satyriasis should undergo medical treatment for the condition, but also that the rooms of his house should be strewn with cold flowers, and herbs and the leaves of cold trees to prevent the heat of passion taking a hold of his body. To keep a man youthful, he should regularly drink a decoction of fennel, which was supposed to make old men seem younger. This was claimed to have been proven by authors and philosophers, who had noticed that old serpents would often go out to eat fennel to become strong, mighty, and young again.

If you were an unscrupulous person and wished to steal someone else's lover, there were herbs to assist you. Placing powdered vervain between the lovers would cause friction, leading them to argue and fall out. A quicker solution for removing an unwanted lover, yours or somebody else's, was easily achieved by poisoning and the chances of being caught were very low, even well into the nineteenth century. Many poisonous plants commonly grow wild in the UK, so there would nearly always be something available. The monk Walafrid Strabo wrote that if you were worried that your stepmother was trying to poison you, you should take a brew of horehound,

Gladden, or the stinking iris, *Iris foetida*, was suggested as a remedy if you had been poisoned.

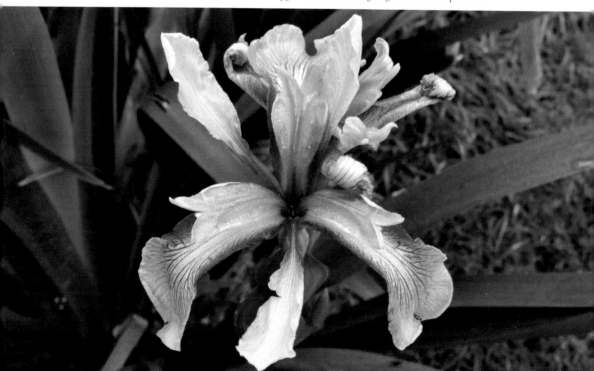

which would even counter the powerful poison of aconite. I personally wouldn't put too much faith in it. Another remedy for poisoning was to take equal quantities of dragons, gladden iris and mint, crush them to a pulp and add them to wine. Warm the wine before drinking it. You would most likely be violently sick after drinking the medicine. If you suspected that you were the person that was about to be poisoned, you may risk taking a, mithridate, a medicine that is given to protect against poisoning by giving increased doses of the poisonous substance.

Sadly, romance is often doomed to fail, so if you were suffering from the loss of a lover, opium poppy could be taken to ease your grief.

If on the other hand, you had wooed, won your true love, and married them, you needed to keep them faithful. To maintain the love between man and wife, take periwinkle leaves and make them into a powder. Wrap the powder with earthworms and add houseleeks.

If you doubted your wife's fidelity, put marigold, *Calendula*, in a church when your wife enters. If she has been unfaithful, she will be unable to leave until the marigold has been removed. It was claimed that this was both proven and true!

Chastity

Although most of the population probably wanted to induce sexual potency, there was a part of the population that wanted to reduce their sex drive. Over-indulgence was thought to be bad for the eyesight. Venery and lechery, except for the conception of children, were sinful, even within marriage. For those in holy orders who had taken vows of chastity, namely clerics, nuns, anchorites and hermits, lust, in thought or deed, was to be avoided. There were several plants that were thought to assist chastity. The most famous was *agnus castus*. The name is thought to derive from *Agnus Christi*, meaning, the Lamb of God. It was especially beneficial for those who had taken vows of chastity because the plant was said to make both men and women chaste. The classical author Thracolidon said that it, 'destroys the foul lust of lechery.' Some people simply lay the plant on their body, others ate it before they went to sleep in the hope that this would prevent what we may now call wet dreams, but which medieval men considered to be the outcome of a devil-sent female spirit known as a succubus. This female sprit would visit the man at night and tempt him to break his vows either within a dream, or as a result of masturbation. Consorting with a succubus would also destroy the moisture of a man's seed and prevent conception with a mortal woman. Women did not escape temptation as they suffered from the visitations of male demons known as incubi.

In Britain, the true *agnus castus* is often killed by a severe frost, so the hardier tutsan, *Hypericum androsaemum*, could be grown instead, as it was said to have similar properties. Tutsan is a medium sized shrub with yellow flowers. The berries begin with a yellow colour, turning red, then black as they ripen. The plant grows naturally in woods and dry ground, but it is tolerant of many situations. One writer said there are many species of Tutsan, which suggests that he considered all the *Hypericum* genus to have the same properties. It was best to eat the root roasted or boiled, as if it was eaten raw it could induce headaches, which some would say helps to preserve chastity anyway.

Another cure for lechery was to pulverise nettle seeds and pepper, then mix the powder with honey or wine. This was apparently so effective that if you gave it to a dog that was chasing a bitch on heat, the dog would abandon her, and she would go mad!

If a woman wanted a quiet night's sleep, she could a mix a powder of fennel seed in sweet wine and give it to her partner, so the man would not be stirred to lustful thoughts. A plaster of hemlock laid on the pubic area quenches lechery and the flow of semen.

More pleasant was the use of the cold virtues of roses to quell the heat of passion, so that sugar or syrup of roses were said to greatly reduce desire and could easily be added to food. The juice of leeks was another cure for lechery in men and women, although another source suggests that they would have a contrary effect! As leeks were readily available for most of the year, it makes one wonder at how common lechery was when a large proportion of the population ate leeks regularly.

Those who had taken vows of chastity had much to fear if they broke them. (Getty Images)

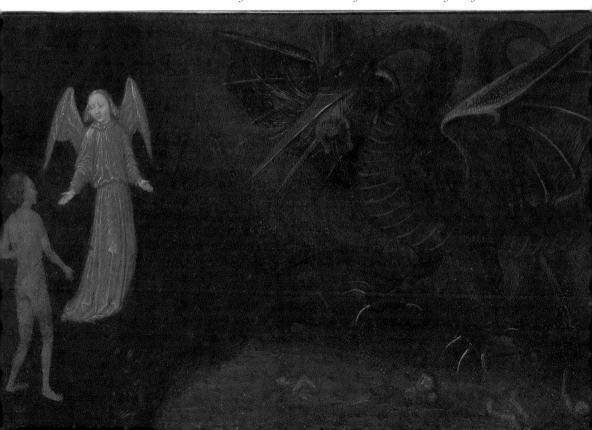

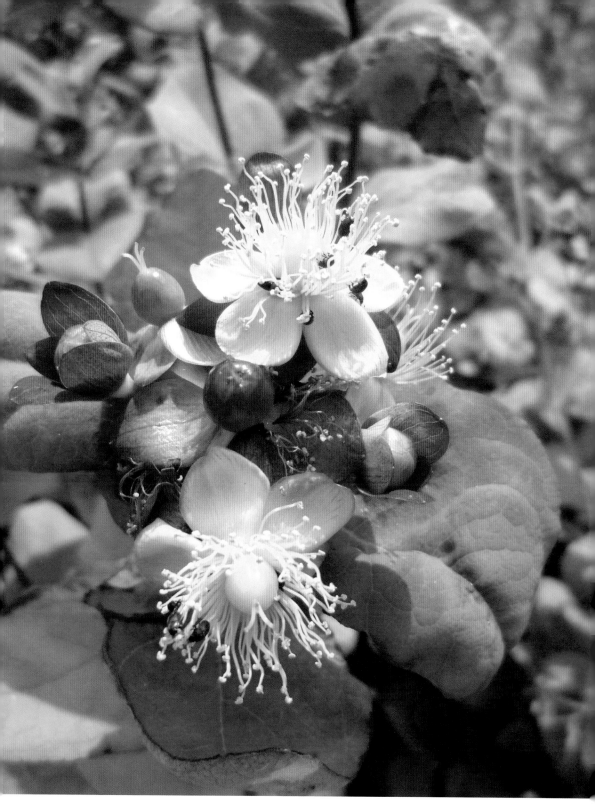

Tutsan, the English Agnus Castus.

CHAPTER 9

Childbirth, Babies and Nursemaids

Gynaecological and obstetrical problems were often referred to ambiguously, which is hardly surprising considering that the authors were mostly male and had taken religious orders.

Once married, a woman was expected to conceive and produce healthy children. Ginger was an aid to conception, but only for the wealthy as it was expensive. Motherwort, *Artemisia vulgaris*, is a common plant of roadsides, hedges and waste ground. This common, and now largely ignored, plant was once known as the mother of all herbs, or simply motherwort. It was used as a herb for female problems and was a freely available aid to conception, as was *Leonorus cardiaca*, another plant known as motherwort which was introduced into Britain in the late medieval period. According to the Bible and some of the herbals, mandrake would help to increase female fertility and aid conception, but it was not always readily available and was very expensive to buy. Most herbals warned that mandrake was a very cold plant, with great strength and that taking too much would kill you. A more enjoyable means for a woman to conceive was for her to eat a trout cooked in goat's milk prior to intercourse. Usually, any failure of conception was placed on the woman, but the *Trotula* proposed the original and generally controversial idea, that both men and women could be at fault when children were not conceived. If a couple were unable to conceive but were unsure whose fault this was, they could both urinate into separate earthenware pots that had not yet been used. In each pot they should stir in some wheat bran to slightly thicken the liquid. The pots should be clearly marked so that it would be easy to tell them apart. The pots were then to be stored somewhere safe for ten days and ten nights. If the woman was at fault, her pot would be found to contain worms, and vice versa. If there were no worms, then the couple would conceive, but only when God wills it.

Conception conception was a good start, but preferably the baby should be a boy. There were herbs with the property to help to select the desired sex of a baby. Orchids were a popular aphrodisiac and quite safe compared to most of the others, with the

MEDIEVAL PLANTS AND THEIR USES

added advantage that they could be used to help select the sex of a baby. The roots of an orchid are divided into two nodules, similar to testicles, leading to orchids being given more vulgar names, such as dog or fox testicles. One half of the orchid root is usually larger than the other. If the couple wanted a boy, the man should eat the larger piece before intercourse. If the woman conceived, the baby would be a boy. If the woman ate the smaller part and conceived, the child was likely to be a girl, with the odds equally are good in either case. A drink made of teasels was also thought to help a woman conceive a boy.

Throughout history, until fairly recently in the western world, giving birth was the most dangerous thing a woman could do. No matter how wealthy you were, the chances of dying because of pregnancy or childbirth were very high, and with few safely reliable methods of controlling fertility, women could spend much of their child-bearing age being pregnant. There were numerous plants that were said to help make the birth easier yet there was usually a serious risk to the health of the woman as many were toxic, such as birthwort, *Aristolochia*.

Horehound could be taken to shorten a woman's pregnancy and it would relieve a bad cough too. One of the safer recipes to ensure that a woman with child delivered and bear her child easily was to drink the juice of balsamita and water mint simmered with wine. The seeds of the corncockle could be burned, because fumes were thought to assist a woman to give birth without harm or peril. A drink made of catmint would help to ease childbirth, which may have helped as modern herbalists still advise that a pregnant woman should not eat catmint because of the risks. If the baby had died in the womb, there were many plants that were thought to help remove the foetus. Making a pessary of mallow mixed with goose grease, or alternatively the root of the stinking iris mixed with honey, and then inserting it into the vagina was considered a safe option for the

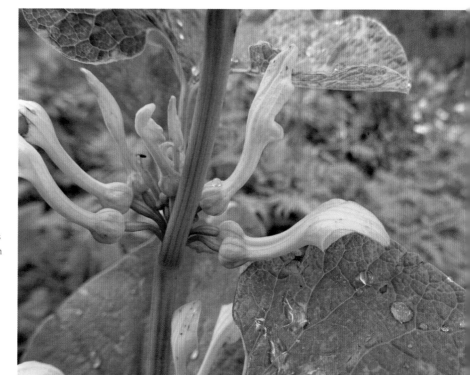

Aristolochia was one of the plants used to help with childbirth.

mother. Cabbage seeds, elecampane, parsley and centaury were other suggestions for ingredients. Boiling a quantity of garlic in its skin and then bathing the mother for some time was said to be useful. One writer noted that caraway delivers, and quickly, with the bonus that it has a very likeable scent and flavour.

Once the baby had been safely delivered, it was placed in a cradle surrounded by fern fronds to deter the devil and keep the baby safe from evil.

Producing enough milk for a baby could be difficult for a mother who had a poor diet. There were many suggestions to increase milk production. Regularly drinking a decoction of anise would ensure that the mother or wet-nurse would produce enough milk. The milky sap of lettuce resembles milk, so it was thought to increase the milk in women, and similarly to be helpful for the production of seed in men. Mary's thistle, *Silybum marianum*, has white marking on the veins of the leaves which were supposed to represent the milk of the Virgin Mary and were thought to help the wet nurse to produce milk.

If the woman's milk was thought to be stuck or curdled in her breasts, she should cook small bundles of mint stems in wine and oil, then place them as a plaster on her breasts.

When the time came to wean the child from the breast, the mother or nurse's nipple could be washed with a solution of the bitter-tasting wormwood to discourage the baby from suckling. Freshly crushed hemlock laid on the mother's or wet nurse's breasts would help her milk production to stop.

Hanging a daffodil bulb around the neck of a child when they were teething would reduce their pain and stop them crying. If a fractious child would not go to sleep, the women of Salerno had an answer. They would give their children powdered white poppy mixed into their milk. There was a warning that you must be careful to make sure that it was the white poppy seed; if you gave the child black poppy by mistake, it would be fatal. A tea made of poppy heads was another way to send a child to sleep. Older children were more likely to be, 'chastised and beaten on the bare buttocks and loins,' with birch twigs if they misbehaved.

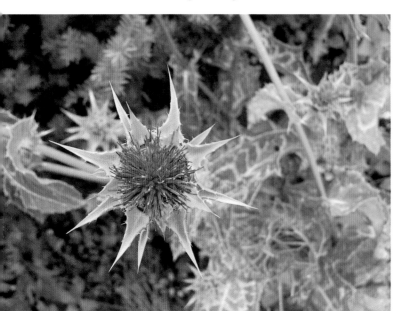

Left: The white markings on the leaves of Mary's thistle represented the milk of the Virgin Mary.

Opposite: Hemlock could be used by women to stop the production of breast milk.

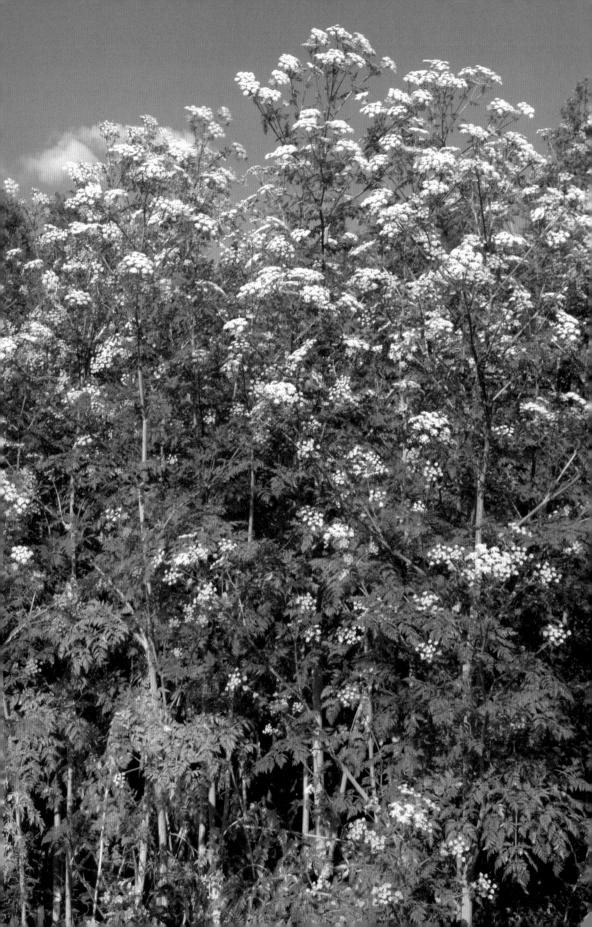

CHAPTER 10

Clothing, Laundry and other Household Tips

L inen was the material for making under garments. It is easy to wash clean and dry it, unlike the wool cloth worn by many of the general population, or the finer materials worn by the wealthy. Linen is made from the stem fibres of flax, *Linum usitatissimum*. The pale blue flowers of flax may be seen growing in the UK, but now it is for the seed, from which linseed oil is extracted, rather than for the fibres. The process for obtaining the fibres required a lot of labour. The ripe stems would first be hand-pulled from the ground to ensure the maximum length of the fibres. The stems would be bundled and dried. When dry, the flax would be retted, to soften the outer casing of the stems, either by lying the bundles on dew-soaked grass or placing them in slowly running, shallow water.

Harvested flax stems.

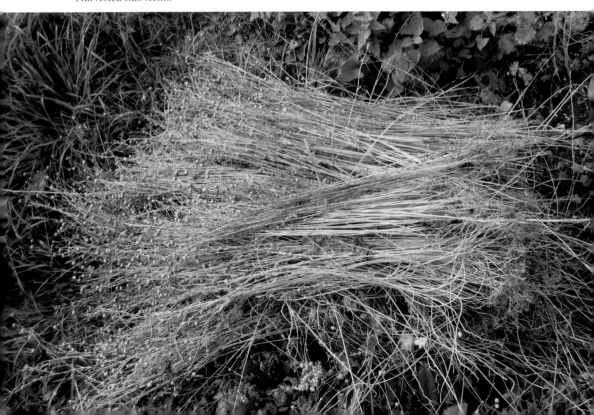

A flax breaker would crush the outer covering of the stems which would then be thrashed against a bed of spikes to remove the casing to leave the fibres which could be combed ready for spinning. The best fibres are a soft golden colour. It was not for nothing that ladies were often described as having flaxen hair. Spinning was a woman's work. Many pictures show women using a drop spindle as they rest or walk. By the late fourteenth century, spinning wheels were available for those that could afford them, but they were not very labour saving as recent experiments suggest a woman could walk up to twenty miles a day walking to and away from a spinning wheel to spin her thread. Processing flax may have been time consuming, but the spun thread had many uses. Fishermen used it to make sails. Linen nets were used for fishing and hunting. Archers used linen bowstrings. Lines of flax were used to measure land. Purses, bags and sacks could be made using linen.

The stems of hemp were treated in much the same way as flax to extract the fibres. Records for Norwich cathedral in 1429-30 tell us that surplus hemp was sold for 4s.

Once spun, the thread could be used for sewing or to be woven into cloth. Clothing was expensive because it took such a long time to produce, even from the cheaper materials.

To wash the clothing, soapwort, *Saponaria officinalis*, was much preferable for fine fabrics. Soap was made of animal fats and lye. If the soap had not matured properly, it could still be very caustic and could damage material and skin. The roots of soapwort could be dug up in the autumn and dried for later use. The stems and leaves produce the soap too but produce green suds because of the chlorophyll they contain.

Hemp was grown for its fibres and medicinal use.

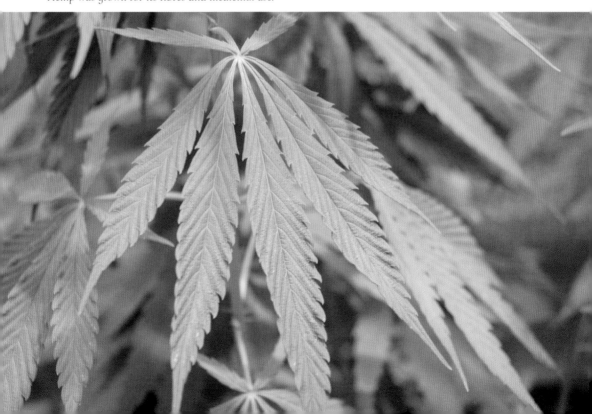

The root pieces could be tied in linen bags and added to the washing water. Soapwort spreads rapidly by roots and seed, so a plentiful supply is easy to maintain.

The outer layer of clothing was usually made of wool. To make the wool cloth thicker, it went through a process known as fulling. This could be treading the cloth in vats of urine, but it could also be brushed to raise the nap for a velvet-like effect. The brushes were made using the seed heads of the fullers' teasel. This is similar to the teasel that is found growing wild which has lilac flowers. The fuller's teasel is quickly identified by its white flowers and the head has a more rounded seed case. There is another important difference. The seed heads of the fuller's teasel are shorter and stubbier, similar in effect to a stiff wire brush, but much gentler to the cloth. The heads were collected when they were dry, then set in a frame to make a brush. The brushes continued into use well into the twentieth century when they were set onto rollers for the best mohair sweaters and the cloth used to make the green baize for the best snooker and billiard tables.

With much of the clothing made of wool, it was tempting to the common clothes moth, *Tineola bisselliella*, whose larvae happily gorge on the fibres of wool, skins, fur and feathers. To deter the moths from laying their eggs, bags of dried wormwood leaves could be added to the clothes chest or cupboard amongst the clothing. Edward IV's Wardrobe Accounts

Soapwort produces suds that will clean cloth.

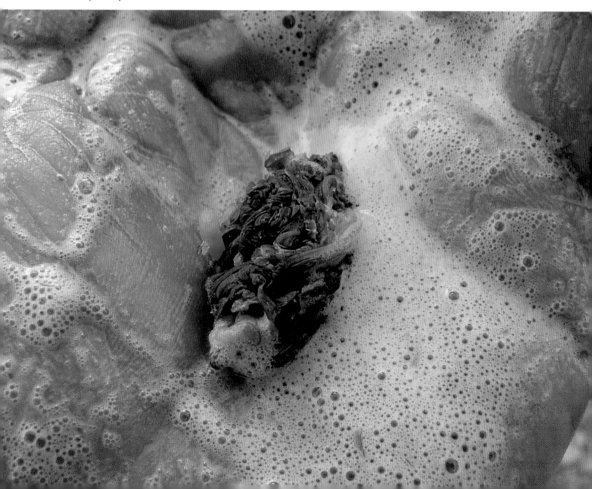

record bags of fustian stuffed with anneys (aniseed) and ireos (iris) being placed between the linen to deter insect pests. Regular brushing and exposing the clothing to hot sun would also help, although the sun option may have caused the colours to fade.

To add a slight perfume to clothing, having a similar effect to a modern wash, bags of dried scented herbs could be included. Dried rose petals that had been sifted to remove any bugs could be spread over clothing. Powdered orris root has a slightly violet scent and is still used as a fixative to help preserve the scent of other plants in perfumes or potpourri. Bed linen and clothing could be dusted with powdered orris to give a pleasant smell. Orris roots could be used as a starch for linen. To make it, dig up a third of the older roots of orris plants in the autumn. Peel the roots, cut them into thin disks and thread them onto a cord which should be hung in the sun until the roots are thoroughly dry. The dried disks are made into a fine powder by pounding them.

To ensure ownership of your linen, perhaps in case of a dispute if somebody attempted steal your washing, it was suggested that you should stamp your linen with your mark. Obtain some of the black axle grease from a cart, adding ink, oil and vinegar. Boil them together. Warm your stamp, dip it in the mix and stamp your cloth. Wooden stamps were often used to make patterns on cloth for wall hangings, so they were easy to make or buy.

A Fuller's Teasel Brush.

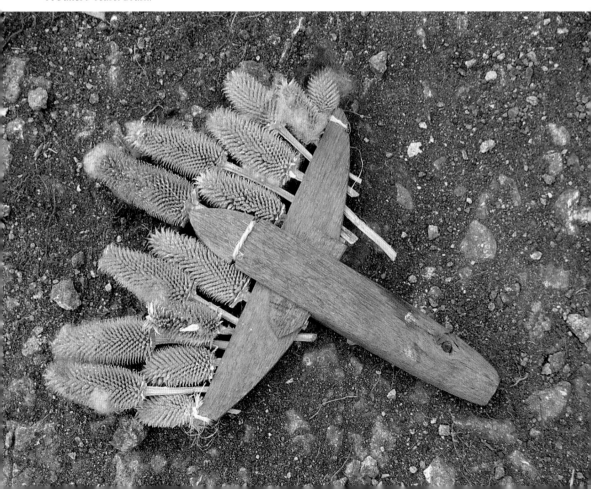

Removing grease and marks caused by accidental spills of food must have been common and there were methods for removing them. Dabbing warm wine, presumably white if it is put on paler clothing, and leaving it for two days was said to lift out grease.

Lye and wood ash were rubbed onto cloth to remove stains and it was even said to restore faded colours. The Ménagier of Paris said that he had heard that rubbing verjuice – soured fruit juice – whether old or new, was equally as good as lye for removing stains. He mentions that some people even claimed the verjuice would restore the colour of cloth, but he personally did not think that this would work.

To keep the floors of the house clean, you needed a good besom broom. Brooms were easy to make and would use the materials available locally, so the broom plant, *Cytisus scoparius*, was not the only plant material used to make the head, heather was used if it grew locally. The twigs of birch made very good besoms, 'to sweep and to clean houses of dust and of other uncleanness,' noted one writer. If you needed a stiff brush, the stems of butcher's broom, *Ruscus aculeatus*, with their prickly cladodes, (they have the appearance of leaves) are very effective. A sheaf of the stems can be bound together

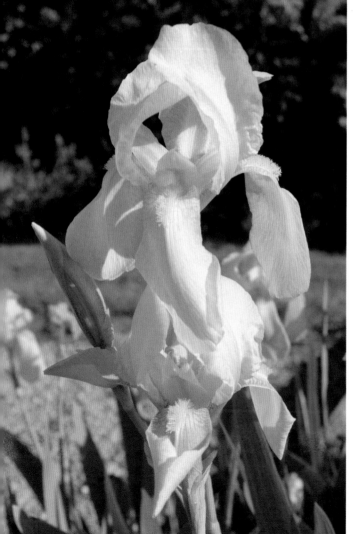

with a strip of willow bark or a withy to make a hand brush or bind the stems to a longer pole to make a broom. The broom was associated with women, so it is hardly surprising that witches were often believed to fly upon broomsticks; today they would be flying on the vacuum cleaner.

Poisonous plants were used for practical purpose of killing household pests, and sometimes unwanted rivals. Flies in the house were certainly not desirable. To get rid of them, you could cut pieces of the poisonous red and white toadstool, Fly Agaric, and place them in a bowl of milk. Attracted by the sweet liquid, the flies drink and then die.

The dried roots of orris, *Iris florentina*, could be used to starch linen.

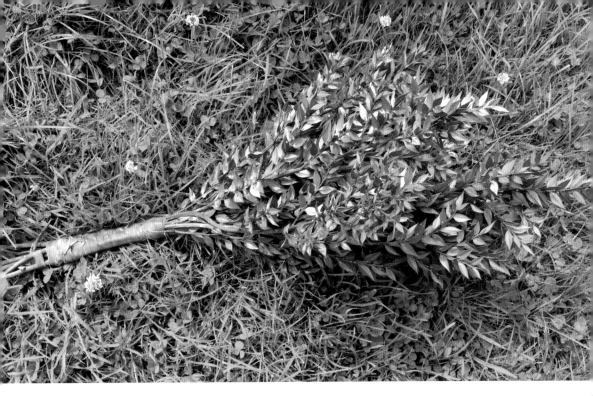

Above: Butcher's broom stems bound with willow bark to make a hand brush.

Right: Fly agaric was used to kill flies.

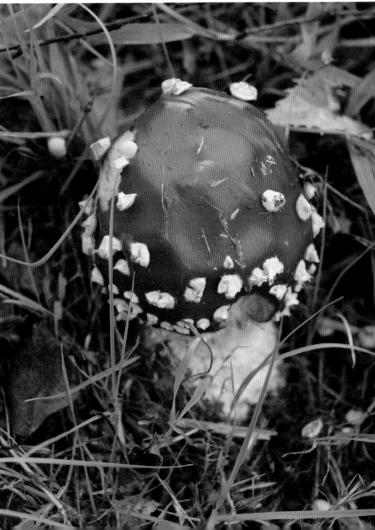

Another way of destroying flies was to mix powdered corncockle seed with honey and smear it on the wall. The flies eat the honey and then die. Powdered hellebore root in honey was a good alternative. Several manuscripts describe how to prepare *Aconitum napellus*, often known as monkshood, to kill mice and rats by pounding the roots together with breadcrumbs. Hellebore could be used in a similar fashion to kill household vermin. Monkshood has another name, wolf's bane, because it could be used to kill wolves when mixed in larger quantities with meat which would be left out for the wolves to eat. If you were more energetic and preferred to hunt for the wolves, the juice of wolf's bane could be rubbed onto arrowheads, so even if the wolf was only wounded by an arrow, it would die later from poisoning. In 1281, Edward I declared that wolves must be hunted to extinction, and this happened in the south but it is believed they lasted until the late fourteenth century in Yorkshire, wolf's bane or not!

The sea squill, *Urginea maritima*, was mentioned in Charlemagne's plant list as *Scilla-de-morts-aux-rats*, because the bulb was well-known as a rat poison.

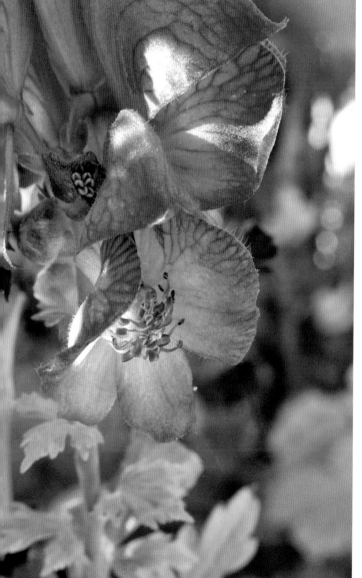

Many medieval books warned of the dangers of eating the wrong sort of fungi. Poisoning from eating a poisonous toadstool, accidental or otherwise, still happens. Most will give you a bad case of diarrhoea and stomach cramps. Unfortunately, some are fatal, and even today there is still no antidote for the poison of the Destroying Angel. Because of the dangers from eating the wrong type of fungi, they do not appear in many medieval recipes, but if you had inadvertently poisoned yourself, wormwood taken with hot water and vinegar was known as an antidote. If you had no wormwood, mustard seed would do the job.

Aconitum napellus, Monkshood, was used to poison pests.

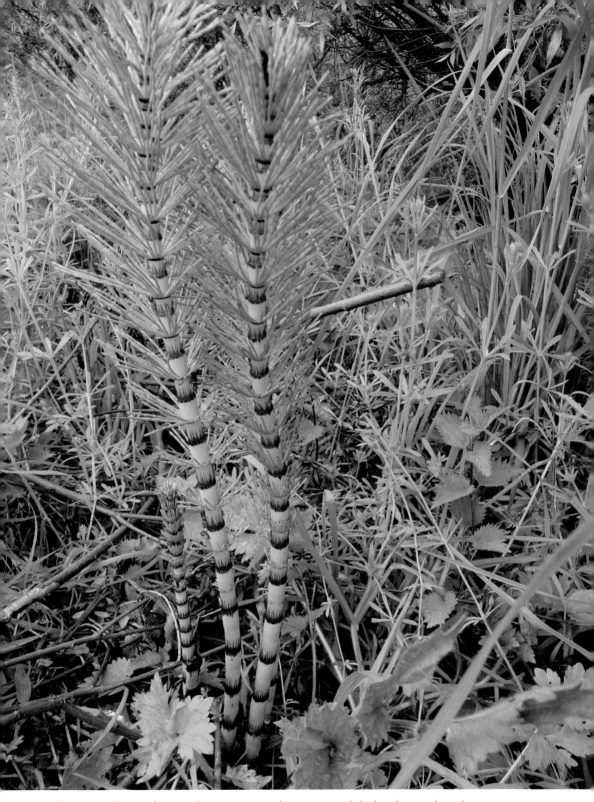

Shavegrass or horsetail was used to scour pots and pans, or to polish glass, horn and wood.

To give a good shine to your possessions you needed horsetail, *Equisetum*, which was known as shavegrass. It prefers to grow in the same moist habitat as rushes. Horsetail has a knobbly stem which can be pulled apart into small sections, as was noted by a medieval writer. Each section has a circle of leaves around the perimeter, giving the appearance of a chimney sweep's brush. The stems were to be harvested in the summer and dried. The dried stems can then be burned, and the ashes stored in bags or boxes to use as a polishing powder. The powder, or the dried and fresh stems were used to, 'polish combs, bowls and cups.' The plant has a high silica content, making it an excellent polish for use on bone, gesso, glass, horn, metal cooking pots, weapons and armour and wood.

Lighting

Beeswax was expensive, so many people could not afford to use candles very often, if at all. Instead, lighting came from bowls of oil or fat with a wick, or a rushlight in a holder. The best rush to make rush lights is *Juncus effusus*. It has a round section. One herbal called the rush 'paper, that is to say food for the pyre, or food for the fire, because, when it is dry, it is the most suitable to nurture the fire in lamps.'

The author went on to describe the rush as a pretty plant that has very white marrow that is like a sponge. To prepare a rushlight, cut the rush in late summer or autumn as long as possible. Then cut into lengths of 30 cm or so, which should burn for

Peeling the rush to reveal the spongy interior.

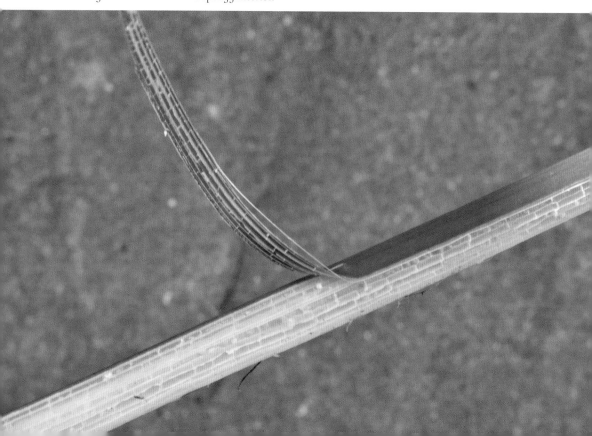

fifteen minutes, but may last longer. Carefully peel off the green outer casing using a thumb nail or a sharp knife; but leave a thin strip of the casing along the full length of the section to give it strength. The less that remains of the bark, the more clearly it will burn whether as the wick of a lamp or as a rushlight.

Lay the rushes in the sun until they are thoroughly dry. Any type of available animal or bird fat can then be melted over a low heat and the sections of rush put in the pan until the grease is soaked into the pith. Dry the rush pieces and store them somewhere out of the way of rats, mice and animals that may be tempted to eat them. The rush is set at about 45 degrees in a metal holder that is like a pincer, or you can use a piece of split wood. The rush can be used as wicks for fat or oil lamps. Unlike candles, rushlights are easy to burn at both ends, but there still won't be much light!

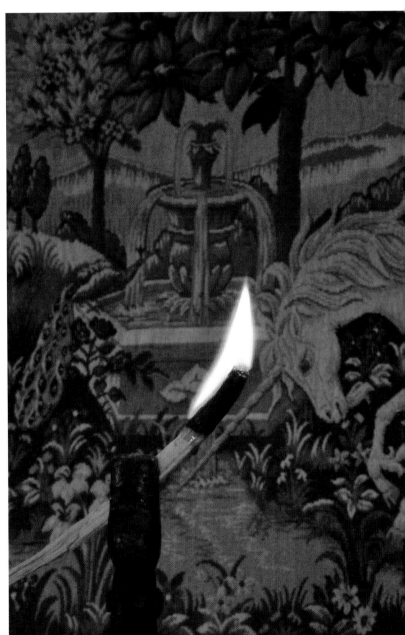

Rushlights burned quickly
and gave off little light.

Strewing

Scenting the air was important during the medieval period. Diseases were thought to be spread by bad air which could come from many sources. According to the fourteenth century *Litil Bok of the Pestilence*, to remain healthy, it was desirable 'therefore, as much as to them is possible, it is to eschewe every cause of putrefaction and stinking ... every foule stycnhe is to be eschewed, of stabyl, stinking feldys, wayes or stretes.'

Water from gutters and storage tanks was likely to become corrupt and stinking. Even the kitchen odours were not exempt, for 'where the wurtys and cooles putrefyed it maketh a noysful savour and stynkyng.'

Pleasant smells were beneficial for health. Sweet odours would banish foul stenches or purify the air, making it healthy again. 'For in lyke wyse as by the swete odour of bawme (Lemon Balm) the herte and the spyrites have recreation, so of evyl savours they be made feble ... Let your hous be made with fumigacion of herbes, that ys to saye with leuys of baye tree.'

Dishes of sweetly scented petals and leaves could be kept in rooms to give them a pleasant atmosphere. Rose, or other scented petals or aromatic leaves should be

Dried rose petals were used to scent rooms.

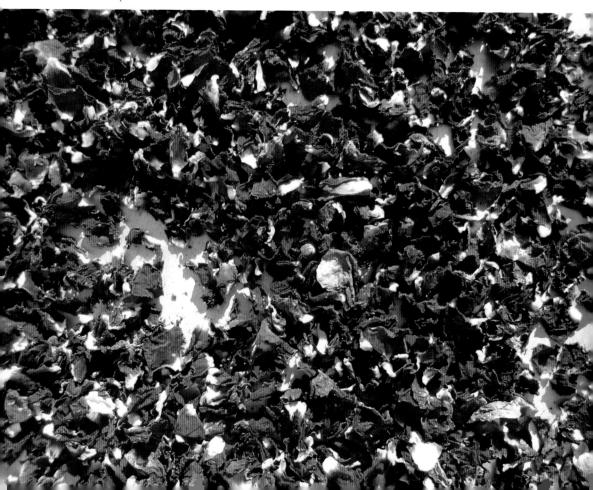

picked once the dew was dry. They were spread on cloths or trays and set out in the in the sun to dry. Turning regularly ensured the petals were thoroughly dry. The petals could be placed in decorative bowls throughout the house. Adding some orris powder helped to enhance and preserve the scent. Confusingly, medieval writings often refer to the rose petals as leaves, which has caused some problems in modern attempts to reproduce recipes where people have used the actual leaves rather than the flowers.

You could sprinkle your house with roses, vinegar and pine leaves to scent it and to help to keep it cleansed. A sweetly scented house would be welcoming to guests. Many floors were made of beaten earth or for those with more money, stone slabs. Rushes were spread over the floor, especially during very cold weather, to absorb the wet and mud brought into the house on people's shoes. The other purpose of the rushes was to insulate the feet from the cold floor. Most people usually wore thin-soled shoes indoors, although later medieval pictures often depict finely-decorated pattens to slip over the foot to avoid direct contact with a cold floor. Plants that were thought to deter flies and other unwanted insects, such as fleabane, rue, tansy and wormwood were added to the rushes along with plants with leaves that contained volatile aromatic oils that would release their odour as people trod on them, such as rosemary, thyme and lavender.

There were other scented plants that could be utilised to cover bad odours. Sweet woodruff is a low growing plant with white flowers. The leaves retain a strong smell that resembles new-mown hay, which would be pleasant inside a house, whether on the floor or in bowls to scent a room, although there was a warning that if you used too much, the overpowering scent could cause headaches. The flowers of sweet

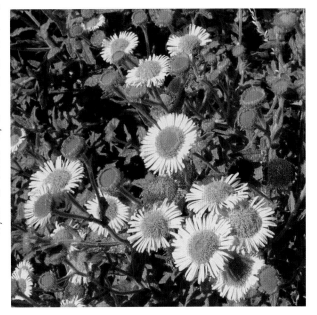

woodruff can be added to white wine to give it a much different flavour. This wine is still popular in Germany where it is known as May wine.

Lice and fleas could be controlled with the leaves of horsemint or by sprinkling water that had been simmered with gorse. If you have fleas on your body, rub your body with rue juice to get rid of them.

Fleabane was useful for strewing on floors or in clothing to deter fleas.

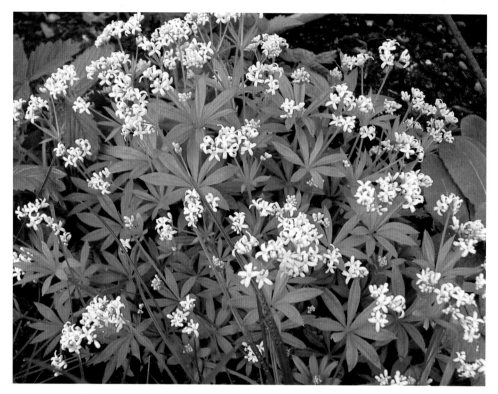

Sweet woodruff has a scent similar to newly mown grass.

In some households the mattress could be stuffed with straw or hay, so strewing herbs could be added to deter fleas and to add a pleasant scent. As the name suggests, lady's bedstraw would be a suitable choice.

The wealthy did not eat banquets as frequently as films suggest, but there were many expectations of the behaviour of the guests at most meals. Washing your hands was a necessity as you shared dishes with other people at your table. Servants would bring you decorated ewers of scented water and cloths to dry your hands before the meal and between courses.

TO MAKE A WATER FOR WASHING HANDS AT MEALS

Boil sage leaves in water. Strain and leave to cool. Use whilst still slightly warm. Other aromatic herbs, such as camomile, rosemary, or bay could be used. Orange peel may be added for a more exotic experience.

One myth of medieval times is that people ate rotting meat, hence the use of expensive spices, to make the food more appetising. The reality is that you would only eat meat that was at its best, unless you were starving and there was no alternative. Spices were expensive. You would impress your guests by flavouring food with spices to show your

MEDIEVAL PLANTS AND THEIR USES

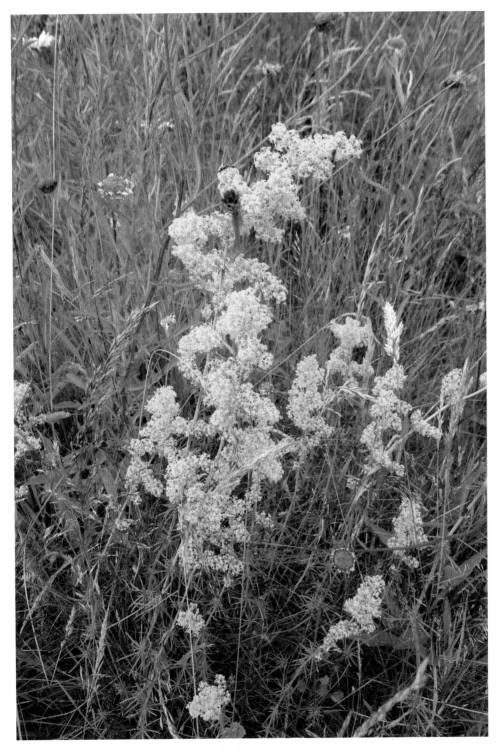

Lady's bedstraw could be used as a strewing herb or added to mattresses and pillow.

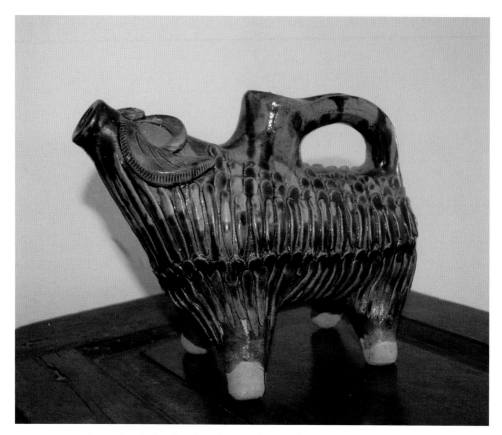

Guests at a meal would wash their hands with scented water from an ewer.

wealth. Another way to make a good impression was to serve wine with the meal, which was certainly affordable for the better-off households, but keeping the wine in a suitable state for drinking was not always easy. If the wine went bad, you could restore it by leaving it outside to be caught by the frost, but if that failed to improve the wine, hanging bags of powdered elder wood with the same quantity of cardamon in the barrel would make a bad-smelling wine good again. If white wine had become a reddish colour, collect a basket full of holly leaves and push them through the bunghole of the barrel and the wine would become white again.

Edible gourds were ingredients for sweet or savoury dishes as they helped to soak up the fat used during cooking, but some gourds had practical uses too as small disposable containers. The dried gourds could be sealed with pitch or beeswax to make containers for wine or water. During the medieval period, gourd-bottles were commonly used to make light-weight water bottles for pilgrims crossing the hot plains of Spain to reach Santiago de Compostela. Saint James, the patron saint of pilgrims, is often shown with a gourd for water hanging from his staff. Henry Daniel grew gourds and commented that pilgrims returning from across the seas often brought

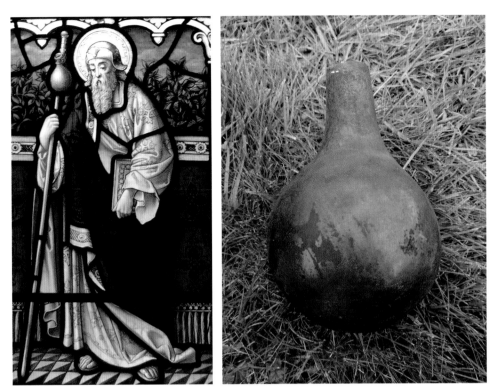

Above left and above right: St James is often shown with a bottle made from a dried gourd.

Below: Verbascum leaves were used medicinally but may have had hygienic uses.

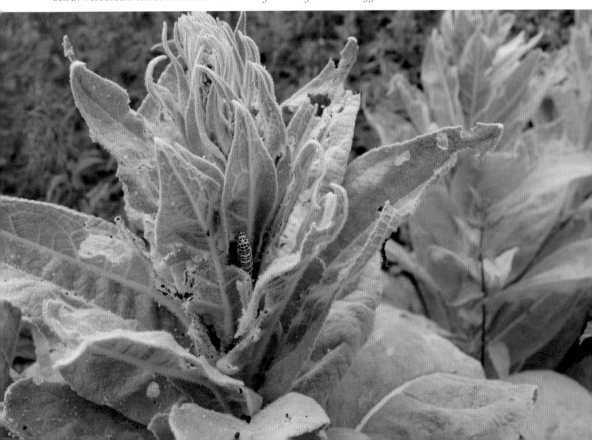

the bottles back from their travels. Daniel suggested hanging gourds in a bakehouse to dry them thoroughly and make them as hard as possible.

Having eaten your food, your body will at some point expel it. Little is recorded about cleaning yourself after using the latrines. Scraps of cloth have been found in places such as Oslo, but archaeology has discovered that plant material may have been used too. Moss has been found in cesspits from the Viking period at Jorvik and at later medieval sites such as Pevensey castle. Pevensey is surrounded by marshland, where the sphagnum moss grows in abundance, so it could have been used throughout the year. In the countryside you may have used whatever was handy, such as grass and soft leaves. There have been suggestions that large leaves such as mullein, *Verbascum*, foxgloves and docks could have been used, but this would be seasonal.

Literary evidence for the use of leaves comes from *Demaunde Joyeus*, printed by Wynken de Worde in 1511, but translated from an earlier French work. This is said to be the earliest joke/riddle book written in modern English. The twentieth riddle asks, Whiche is the moost cleynelyest lefe among all other leues?' And the answer is, 'It is holly leues for noo body wyll not wype his arse with them.' To which we could also add stinging nettles!

MEDIEVAL PLANTS AND THEIR USES

CHAPTER 11

Dyes, Inks and Paints

Clothing that is not coloured is far too boring for most people, unless there is a strong reason to keep things plain, such as the clothing worn by monks and nuns. The church itself was more than happy for those in its higher echelons to wear bright colours and shimmer with gold and silver threads, all for the glory of God, rather than for the glory of man, in theory at least.

People were expected to know their place in society and clothing was no exception. Sumptuary Laws were passed to restrict the colours and materials that certain levels of society were allowed to wear. The first fully legal controls in England were passed during the reign of Edward III, but the fact that the laws were frequently reintroduced throughout Europe suggests little notice was being taken of them for much of the time.

Home dyeing may have taken place, but dyeing cloth was a major industry. The colour produced by a plant dye can vary with the season of the year the plant was harvested and the condition in which it was grown. Most yarns would have been washed in a mordant that helped to fix the colour permanently so that it would not fade rapidly after a few washes. Mordants may affect the final colour of the dye solution. Urine, a waste product, was readily available as mordant. Alum, a mineral salt, is a very good mordant, but it was fairly expensive as it had to be imported into Britain throughout the medieval period. The final colour of the cloth is also affected by the vessel that is used to process dye; iron containers will make a colour darker and sometimes make it almost black. Most illuminated manuscripts show large wooden barrels being used as dye vats, which were less likely to react with the dye to help to keep the final colour pure.

The three most important dyes that were used during the medieval period were woad, *Isatis tinctoria*, which used to produce the best blue dye until it was replaced by indigo, *Indigofera tinctoria*, which came from the East Indies; the roots of madder, *Rubia tinctorum*, gave a red/orange colour. Some people will know the reddish colour of madder from the artist's paint that is labelled as Rose Madder, although it is mostly an artificial colour now. The final important plant dye of the medieval period is weld, *Reseda luteola*, which gives a strong yellow. Other plant dyes were used, such as the lichens which produce a range of colours; brown, orange and yellow; but it was the lichens that contain orchil that were most highly valued for the red/purple dye that they produced. These lichens mostly grow in the north of England and Scotland. Onion skins can produce a wide range of colours from yellow, through orange hues to browns. The skins were readily available simply because so many onions were used for cookery.

Woad was such an important part of the economy that in 1205, King John sent a letter from Geddington, Northamptonshire, to let it be known that Henry Costein, John Glare, Oliver Sutton and Robert de Guido were to be allowed without hindrance to bring twelve frails (large baskets) of woad by ship from St Valery at some time during Pentecost. The woad was then to be prepared in vats and made into the dye. Woad is not a plant that is native to Britain and originates in the Middle East. It is a biennial plant of the cabbage family. During its second year, the plant produces masses of yellow flowers that lead to pendulous green seeds that will turn black upon ripening. The leaves taken during the first year produce the best blue pigment. The woad plant is very hungry and quickly strips nutrients from the soil. The indigo extracted from woad is a pigment and has to be processed further to make a dye that will colour cloth. The method of processing the woad to produce the dye was the most complicated of the dyeing methods and required knowledge and experience to obtain the best colour. The harvested leaves were crushed in a mill, formed into large balls and allowed to dry for several weeks until they were thoroughly dry and became hard. When required for dyeing, the balls were made into a fine powder which was moistened with water and made into heaps causing the woad to heat up. The heaps were frequently turned to ensure a thorough fermentation. This could take about two weeks. The woad was then put into the dye vats with wood ash, lime or two-week old urine, which make the liquid alkaline, and was covered with boiling water. The soaking time in warm water could be up to thirty hours. The alkalinity of the liquid had to be maintained, so needed testing. One way was to feel it between your thumb and fingers. A smooth slippery sensation meant that it was still alkaline. This stage could take thirty hours before the cloth could be added. The magical part of the process is that when the cloth is extracted it will be green and turns blue as the dye oxidises. Stronger colours, or other colours entirely could be produced by over-dyeing.

To make your own woad balls, grow as many woad plants as you can. Once the leaves are fairly large in late May or early June, harvest the largest leaves from each plant, leaving the smaller ones to grow large enough to be harvested later in the year. Chop the leaves finely and squash and shape them into balls using your hands. It is best to wear rubber gloves, otherwise the juice will stain your hands for some days. Dry the balls for later use. The balls will shrink by over half as they dry, so make them at least as large as a tennis ball, if not larger. Continue making balls throughout the growing season.

MEDIEVAL PLANTS AND THEIR USES

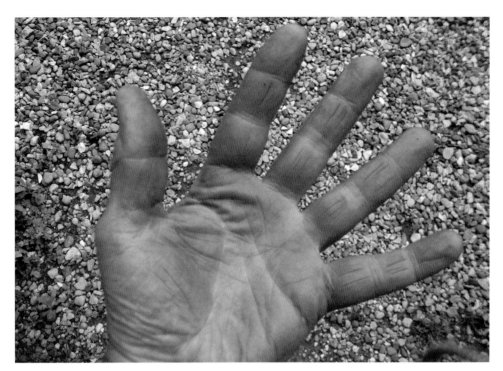

Above and below: Making woad balls stains the skin.

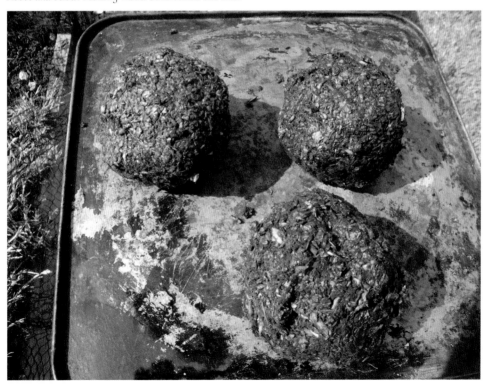

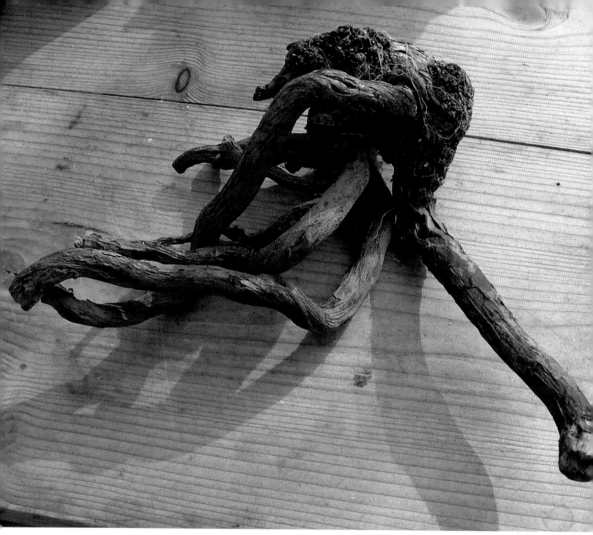

Madder root produces a red dye.

Madder is related to the common goosegrass, except that it is perennial and grows much larger. The roots can be harvested after four or five years and dried. They must be crushed into a powder, the finer the better. The first dye batch will give a strong red/orange colour. Using the dye bath for a second batch of material will give a pretty, dusky pink. It is best not to use an iron pot when using a madder dye. The other main concern is to ensure that the liquid is not allowed to boil, or the dye colour will become brown.

Weld is not a particularly noteworthy plant, and most people would barely notice it growing on the roadside, but it was one on the best plants for producing a yellow dye. The whole plant could be harvested to produce the dye.

Dyers' greenweed is a member of the broom family. It forms a small compact bush and makes a good decorative plant for the modern garden. Despite its common name, the plant produces a yellow dye.

MEDIEVAL PLANTS AND THEIR USES

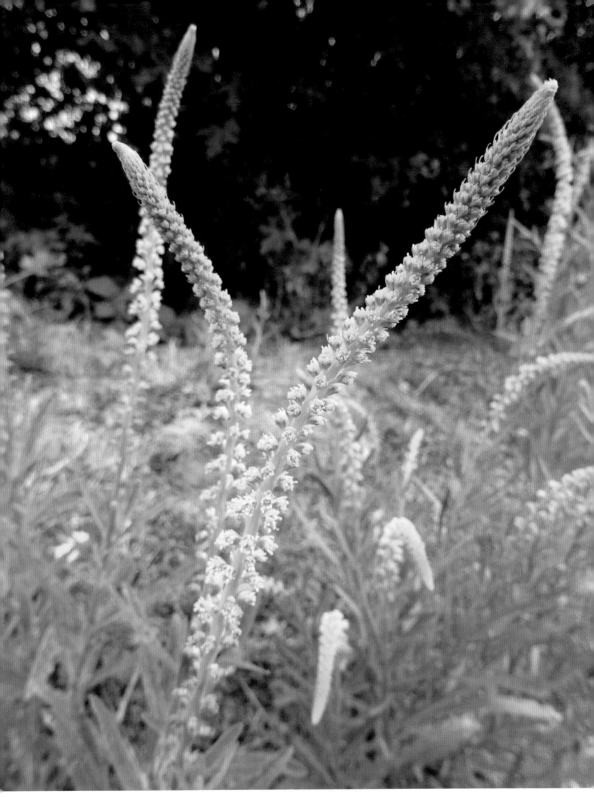

Weld, once a very important dye plant, is now mostly a weed of roadsides and rough ground.

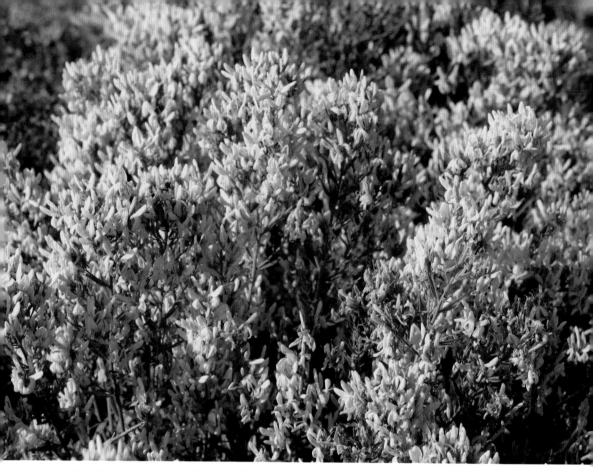

Above: Dyer's greenweed produces a yellow dye.

Opposite: Wormwood was used as a medicine and to deter pests.

Ink would be essential to the running of a large household. Somebody would be needed to record income and expenses, write messages and letters as required and maybe record culinary and medicinal recipes. Most inks were also plant based, although there were many different recipes.

Most documents were written using a black ink, although the church often used red ink to highlight important items. A red ink can be made using madder root, although many coloured inks and paints were based on mineral colours.

Black ink could be made by several methods. Lamp black is produced by holding a piece of metal over a candle flame and scraping off the deposit. Vine branches made into charcoal and then crushed to a powder was another preferred option.

The monk Theophilus, writing c. 1000, gives a recipe that would be perfect for most of western Europe as it relies on using thorn twigs. Which thorn he meant is difficult to say. Blackthorn and hawthorn would be common, and maybe as the method is based on producing charcoal, it may not matter which particular thorn. A process using oak galls and iron filings was another common method for producing black ink.

MEDIEVAL PLANTS AND THEIR USES

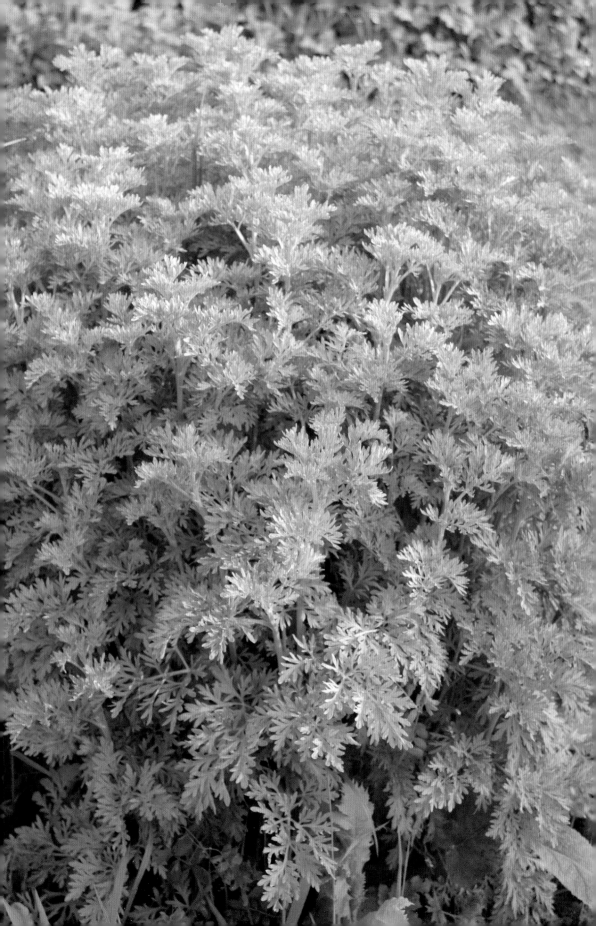

THEOPHILUS' INK RECIPE

Cut thorn branches in spring before the leaves or flowers appear. Tie the twigs in small bundles and leave them to dry in the shade for two to four weeks, then beat them with wooden mallets on a hardwood block to remove the bark. Put the bark in a barrel of water and leave for eight days until the water has absorbed all the sap from the bark. Make several barrels at a time. Remove the water into a clean pan or cauldron and bring to the boil. Add some of the bark to the boiling water to remove any remaining sap. Remove the bark, then add more. Reduce the liquid to a third of the original. Take liquid from the pan, pouring it into a smaller one. Boil until the liquid begins to thicken and turn black. Do not add any water except that which contains sap. When the liquid is thicker, add one third part of pure wine, transferring the mix into two or three new pots. Continue to boil the brew until a skin forms on the surface. Remove the pots from the heat and leave to dry until the black ink purges itself of the red dregs. Make parchment bags with bladders inside (presumably as a waterproof). Pour the pure ink into them and hang the bags in the sun until the ink is thoroughly dry. Use the powder tempered with wine over a low heat and add a little green vitriol, sometimes known as copperas (ferrous sulphate). If the ink is not black enough, heat a piece of iron to red hot and put it into the ink.

Most documents were written on parchment which may be damaged by various pests that would eat it, so scribes could put additives into their inks in the hope of preserving them. To deter pests, you could add something to the ink, as is outlined in this recipe to preserve parchment. 'Let wormwood lie and soak in wine and mix it with your ink and neither mouse nor rat shall gnaw the books that are written in this ink.'

The rituals of the Catholic church were designed to create a sense of the heavenly by flooding the senses of the congregation. There were glittering embroidered vestments, painted walls, and the coloured light pouring through the windows to visually enhance the liturgical drama. The aural senses were enchanted with singing and music. Expensive incense perfumed the air to impart a sense of spirituality into the services, and maybe to reduce the odour of the congregation. Dried plant resins, such as myrrh and frankincense were swung in censers with smouldering charcoal to lead processions, issuing clouds of fragrant smoke. Myrrh was known for its cleansing actions, so this may have been useful as much to protect the clergy as for instilling a sense of otherworldliness in the congregation.

Priests, politicians, and others who relied on their voice as a part of their daily life, could drink a julep of mint to clear roughness of a hoarse voice and give it a clear tone. Liquorice had been used by Roman orators before they were due to give a speech to ensure a clear voice.

  MEDIEVAL PLANTS AND THEIR USES

CHAPTER 12

Animal Health Care

nimals played a vital part in medieval life. Owning animals provided food and wealth. Nothing much was wasted. Skins were transformed into leather and parchment. Horn and bone were used to make useful goblets, combs and as a decorative inlay. Fats were used for food, greasing cart axles and medical or cosmetic creams. Even blood could be made into blood pudding. Animal care may not have been as good as today but keeping your livestock healthy was a major concern. Animal health relied on some of the same medicines and techniques as were used on people. The four humours applied to animal life too. Animals may be bled or purged to keep them as well as possible. Animals showed your status. The wealthy needed fit, healthy horses for work, hunting, war and play. Hawks and hounds for hunting were costly and much time was dedicated to their care. *The Master of Game*, an early fifteenth-century treatise on hunting, included a section on caring for sick hounds. Madness in dogs, usually rabies, was well-known since antiquity. If the infected dog bit either another dog or a person, both would surely become mad too. If caught in time you may be able to prevent the madness taking hold. Lancing the wound and cupping would help too, a technique that was frequently used on human patients:

> There is another help, for men may make sauce of salt, vinegar and strong garlic pulled and stamped, and nettles together and as hot as it may be suffered to lay upon the bite. And this is a good medicine and a true, for it hath been proved, and every day should it be laid upon the biting twice, as hot as it can be suffered, until the time when it be whole, or else by nine days.

The treatment for the eyes was similar to that used for people as it used the greater celandine with the addition of powdered ginger and pepper. It was to be applied to the hound's eye three times a day, making sure that the hound would not be able to rub its eye. The same remedy was used for horses.

Broken bones were to be supported by four splints which were to be bound in place with linen soaked in egg whites and the animal was to have comfrey and self-heal added to its food to help the bones join together. The hounds were valued, as the chapter ends with the words, 'God forbid that for a little labour or cost of this

A CURE FOR MANGE

Take six pounds of honey and heat it whilst stirring, then allow it to cool, then add a quart of Verdigris. Then bring to the boil, with as much of oil of nuts as of the honey and of water, wherein an herb has been boiled that men call in Latin *Cleoborum*, and in other language Valerian, the which make men sneeze, and put all these things together and mingle them upon the fire, stir them well and allow it to cool. Anoint the hound by the fire or in the sun. Make sure that the hound does not lick himself, for it should do him harm. And unless he be whole at the first time anoint him for eight days until the time that he be healed, for certainly he shall be healed.

medicine, man should see his good kind hound perish, that before hath made him so many comfortable disports at divers times in hunting.'

Even for those who did not hunt, dogs were more than mere pets. They were kept as guards to protect your property by barking to alert of intruders or chasing them off. A thief could silence a guard dog by lacing some bait with coriander, which was thought to be poisonous to dogs. Monkshood would certainly work. If your dog was disturbing you by constantly barking, put the plant hound's tongue under the

Greater celandine was used to treat the eyes of animals and people.

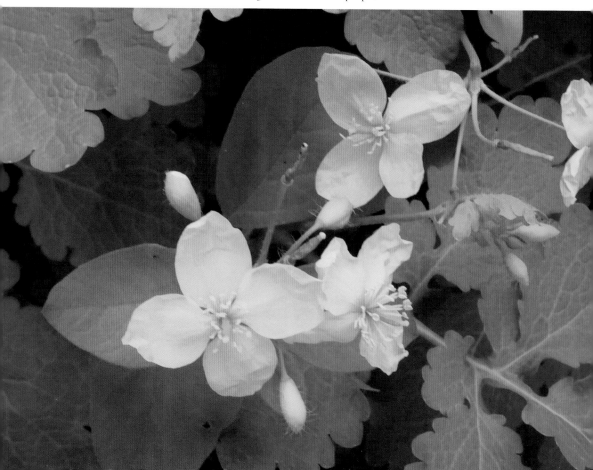

foremost claw and then it will be unable to bark. For those inclined to cruelty to animals, putting hound's tongue in a dog's neck where it cannot remove it was said to cause the dog to turn in frantic circles until it died. This was declared to have been proven to be true by one herbal, as were many other equally dubious claims. Some animals appear to treat themselves by knowing what to eat. Pliny was one of the first people to record that dogs often eat rye grass to make themselves sick.

Sexual desire in animals was something to be encouraged. Owners wanted to increase the numbers of their stock and their profits, so it was desirable to produce healthy lusty males and females that were fertile and receptive. Some of the aphrodisiacs used by people were thought to be equally effective for livestock. To ensure rapid fertility amongst your animals, you must mix the juice of mandrake and teasel and give it to the female animal, and she would soon be pregnant. To maintain healthy livestock the animals needed to be well fed. Sorrel, which commonly grows in grass meadows, was a good food for cattle and other herd animals as it made the beasts stronger and healthy. Clover, although of little use for humans, was another good fodder for cattle.

Sheep were kept for their wool, milk and meat. They could be fattened on lungwort leaves without any noticeable effect on the quality of their milk. Not all plants growing in the wild were safe for grazing animals. Field crocus, sometimes called the autumn crocus, *Colchicum autumnale*, has purple crocus-like flowers in the autumn, with the fleshy leaves appearing during spring. It was known that eating the leaves or corms could be fatal for humans, but there were warnings that if grazing animals ate the leaves they may become weaker, even if they did not die.

When you were moving animals from one place to another there was the risk of them wandering off. If you made a posy of wild celery and tied it around the neck of an ox, the animal would follow you wherever you went.

Bees were an important part of the medieval economy. They produced honey, the main sweetener of earlier times, and the wax honeycomb that was used to make candles and mixed with hot oil to make creams for cosmetics, medicine, polish and sealing wax. Since ancient times, bees were thought to adore the scent of balm, *Melissa officinalis*. Rubbing the leaves onto the hives would encourage the bees to return to it. If you were stung by bees, rubbing the juice of houseleek would ease the pain, but you would have been better to rub the juice of mallow on your skin, as that was believed to prevent the bees stinging you in the first place.

Poultry provided meat and eggs. Galingale fed to geese would ensure that they would lay marvellous eggs, and yew seeds could be fed to hens to encourage egg-laying.

If you wanted a quick and easy method of catching fish, crush the round leaves of birthwort with lime and scatter the mixture on the water, and it would soon kill the fish which could then be collected. It must have been effective as it was written that some people called the substance 'poison of the earth'.

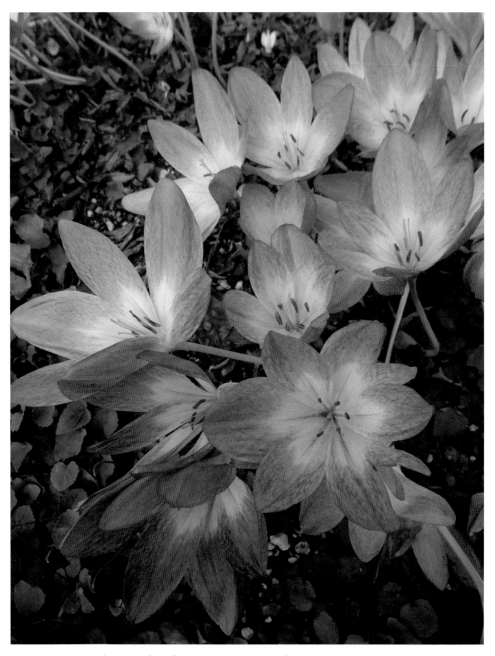

Autumn crocus was known to be a danger to grazing animals.

Snakes cause undue fear in many people. The dread of being bitten by a snake led people to try many methods to deter them. The smoke of burning catmint was thought to repel or drive away adders and all venomous beasts. If you had found a snake, you were to make a garland of fresh betony and place it around the snake. The snake would

MEDIEVAL PLANTS AND THEIR USES

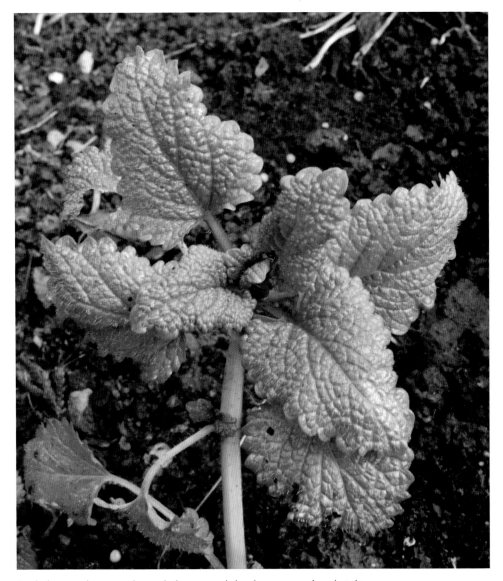

Bee balm, now known as lemon balm, ensured that bees returned to their hive.

be unable to cross the leaves unless it tore at itself with its teeth. The outcome of other methods promised little likelihood of success. 'Oregano juice can be mixed with onions and roses and set in the sun in a brass pot for 40 days when Sirius shines. Place this under your bed, and it will drive away all noxious beasts... as men say.'

The stems of the dragon plant, *Dracunculus vulgaris*, are mottled and were thought to resemble snakeskin, so according to the Doctrine of Signatures they were useful to counter snake bites. You would be safe from the risk of snakebite if you rubbed your hands with the juice from the roots of the dragon plant. This would enable you

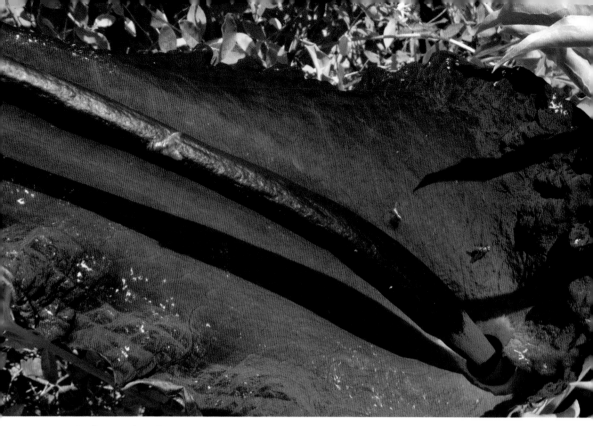

The flowers of the dragon plant produce a powerful stench to attract flies.

to handle adders without risk of being bitten. Rubbing the juice over your body was even better. If the adder did bite you, a potion made of dragons would prevent you from dying. The juice can cause blistering of the skin, so it is preferable to use garlic in much the same way. The dragon name is probably because the flower emits an odour of rotting meat to attract pollinating flies. The breath of the dragon truly stinks!

CHAPTER 13

Harvesting and Preserving Plant Material

All parts of plants were collected and preserved for food and medicinal use, the roots, stems, bark, leaves, flowers and seeds. To obtain the greatest virtue from the herbs they had to be collected at the most beneficial time and often in a prescribed manner. Each part of the plant may be more potent at different times of the year, and as result would need to be gathered when it was at its prime and preserved for later use. Many herbs were considered best used fresh if they were in season, such as the leaves of avens, *Geum urbanum*, which were the most medicinal part of the plant and possessing the best virtue when they were fresh.

General guidelines for harvesting herbs were much the same as for now. Seeds were to be collected when they were fully ripe, and the moisture had dried out somewhat. Flowers were picked when they had just opened, but not when they were faded or withered. Stems were best cut when they were full of moisture before they began to dry and shrink. Roots were usually dug up when the leaves had fallen, generally in late summer or during the autumn, when the root had stored as much energy as possible so that it could survive through its dormant period, which in most of western Europe is usually the winter. Fruits were to be collected when they were at their fullest size before they dropped. The best fruits were the ones that were the heaviest and densest. Those that were large but light should not be selected. Dry weather was the best time to gather most plants. In the past, the herbs growing wild in the fields were usually considered to be more potent than those growing in the garden. The best wild plants were also thought to grow on the hills, even though they tended to be smaller in size than those that grew on the lower ground. For most herbs there still is an ideal time to harvest them so that they retain the most power and effectiveness, but in past times, it was thought that some generally safe herbs could be harmful if they had been collected at the wrong time. Some of the details of harvesting had been inherited from the Greek and Roman herbals, but later adapted to be more acceptable to the church. Physical purity was sometimes said to be important, so a young child may be specified to pick the plant, whereas an older person had to purify themselves by a period

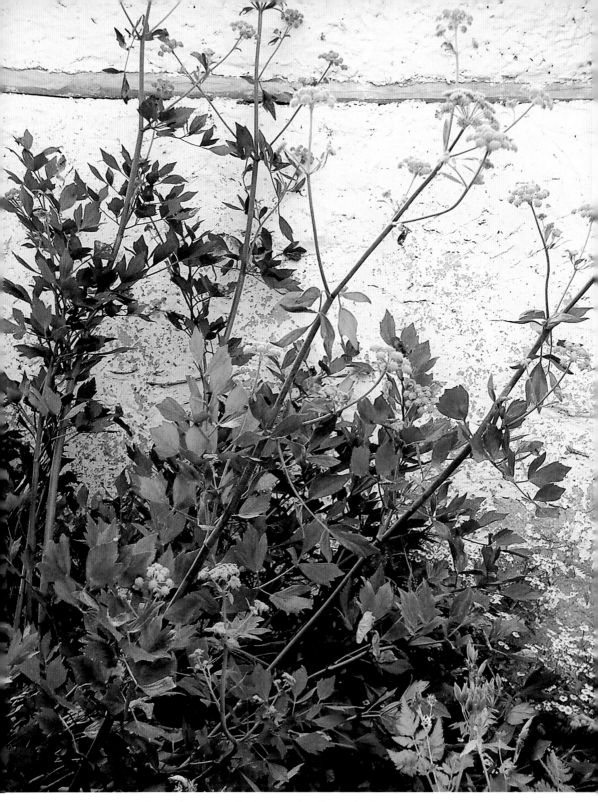

Lovage was used in medicines, as a deodorant and to flavour food.

MEDIEVAL PLANTS AND THEIR USES

of fasting and penitence. Prayers such as the Lord's Prayer and/or the Ave Maria may also be required to ensure that the plant maintained its full medicinal strength when it was taken.

There were dangers to collecting plants. The mandrake is famed for its deathly screams but harvesting other plants could be equally dangerous. Digging up hellebores and peonies was also dangerous as it was thought that a woodpecker would descend out of nowhere and pluck out your eyes. Lovage was a popular food flavouring of the Romans. One early medieval writer, Strabo, wrote that he liked lovage but warned that the scent and juice could cause loss of eyesight. He noted that the seeds were often added to other cures, then disparagingly remarked that the cures were due to the other ingredients anyway. In their favour, the strong celery-flavoured lovage seeds would have covered the taste of less palatable herbs.

It was stressed that some plants should not be dug up and cleaned using anything made of iron or the plant would be rendered useless.

Seasonal tasks and the feast days of saints were good markers for a generally illiterate population as guidance of time for harvesting plants. The valuable, tiny strands of saffron were to be picked before sunrise. *Pedelion*, known as lion's foot or lady's mantle, could be picked whenever it was needed, but preferably after midday. This was so that the dew that frequently rests on the leaves had time to dry. Some herbals suggested that the water from the leaves was supposed to be good for a lady's complexion. Groundsel was another herb that was to be picked after mid-day. Many plants were simply taken whenever they were needed, such as garlic. Walwort, *Sambucus ebulus*, a potent purging plant, was another herb that could be harvested at any time, but only if there had been no rain beforehand.

Sambucus ebulus could be harvested at any time.

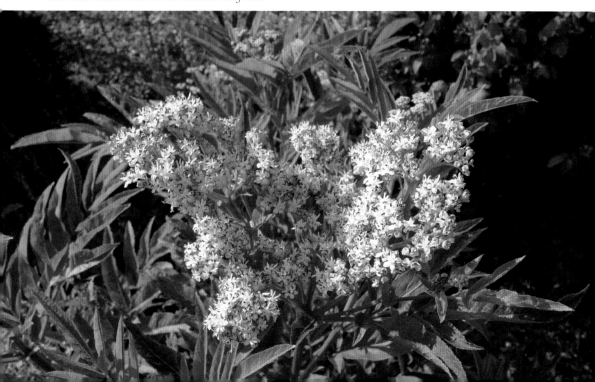

It may be expected that all ferns would all be harvested at the same time of the year, but adder's tongue could be collected in April and again in Lammas, which is in August. Hart's tongue fern was only to be collected in the month of November. The rhizomes of the iris, the fleur de lys, should be gathered at the end of spring. Flowering time was another guide, but this relies on climatic conditions as much as the time of the year. Chamomile was to be gathered in April. This would be before the flowers appear. We now know that a lot of the plant's resources and energy are used to produce flowers and seeds. *Agnus castus*, water calamint, wild garlic and the pink-flowered centaury were to be collected whenever they were in flower.

Most flowers were to be dried in the shade and only held their properties for a year. Rose petals for sugar, syrup of roses and to make oil, were collected during April and May. Rosemary flowers were said to be best harvested during May, although rosemary may flower later in the year, depending on the weather. Galingale, *Cyperus longus*, could be taken at any time of the year, but late spring was thought to be the best time. It was to be dried in the sun for three days and thereafter kept in the shade.

The harvesting of solsicle, *Calendula officinalis*, was very specific. It was only to be gathered on the sixteenth day of June before sunrise, and then only if there had been no rain. Pellitory-on-the-wall was also to be gathered in June before sunrise, whilst pennyroyal could be harvested at any time during the month. Harvest time was recommended as the best time to collect hellebore roots. Fennel seed gathered at the beginning of harvest time would keep for a year, whereas the roots were to be gathered at the beginning of the year and would also keep for a year. The birthworts, *Aristolochia rotunda* and *A. longa* were also best gathered at harvest time. *Pilado*, the root of, *Filipendula*, or dropwort, which was used for medicines, was better if dug from

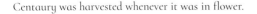
Centaury was harvested whenever it was in flower.

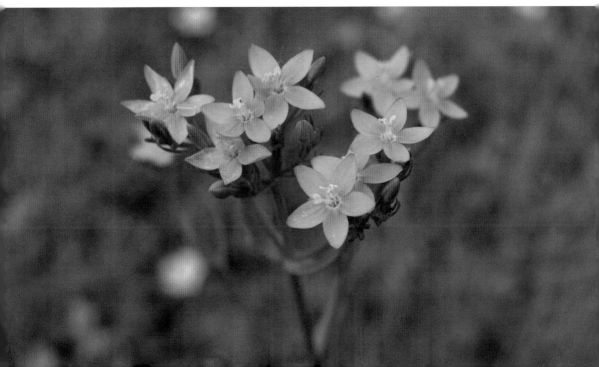

the ground at the end of the harvest. Elderberries for a gout cure were to be collected during the harvest period, between the days of Saint Mary, in other words, the days between the Feast of the Assumption, on the fifteenth of August and that of the Nativity, on the eighth of September. It should be noted that at the time of writing, elderberries in Britain are often still in good condition for picking long after these dates. Ideally, betony was to be gathered in Lammas month, August, when there had been no rain and should be dried in the shade. If it had to be gathered at other times you should gather it before sunrise.

Sometimes the colour of the berries was a guide of the correct time for harvesting. Wild nepe, or white bryony berries were to be gathered when they became yellow, although they are not ripe until they become a dull-red colour. To make a medicinal powder of dried grapes, they should be collected before they were ripe. The moisture was wrung out of them, and the pulp dried in the sun. The dry pulp could then be crushed to a powder that was used with foods to prevent the vomiting that was caused by choleric humours and flux. The root of the gentian, sometimes called baldemayne, according to one herbal, should be gathered at the last end of the year and would keep its potency for up to four years. The root should be yellow inside and feel heavy, a sign that it was solid. You could cut across the root to check that it was not hollow, nor brittle, or powdery inside. The more bitter the taste, the better the medical power.

Some trees exude sap that can be dried. The most well-known ones such as frankincense, myrrh and gum arabic were imported into Europe, although the Europeans, could use *Prunus* species and pine trees for resin. Alternatively, some plants could be pressed to extract the juice, then heated to remove the scum and then reduced to a thick liquid.

The usual advice for the preservation of plants was to dry the material in the sun or in the shade, depending on the particular plant. Most herbal ingredients could be preserved most easily by drying. Once dried, the plants or seeds were best preserved in wooden boxes or cloth bags to protect them from insects and vermin. Another difficulty, especially in poorer households, was preventing dried plants and seeds going mouldy or rotten because of cold and damp buildings.

Fresh roots could be stored in boxes of sand to keep them moist and plump. This was a good way to keep carrots and parsnips over the winter months.

Violet or rose flowers could be made into a sugar by mixing the flowers in a container with ground sugar and sealing the top. Pounding the petals with sugar in a mortar produces something similar to a jam, which will keep for a long period, or you could make a syrup.

A simple rose water can be made by simmering the petals in water, but it will not last for many days. For a more potent liquid, or to make one that lasted longer, you could distil a herb water, which would remove water impurities and hopefully you could keep the water for longer than a few days. For quick use, a water could be brewed like tea, or the plant material left to steep in cold water or wine. Soaking beneficial herbs in wine would produce a tonic wine, which you would drink regularly to maintain your health. Later, herbs would be soaked in a distilled alcohol, such as brandy. Benedictine and Chartreuse were originally drunk as tonics to keep you healthy, rather than for pure pleasure.

If you distilled a herbal wine, you would effectively have a spirit alcohol base that would keep for some years. To distil you would need an alembic, developed by the Arabs. **N.B. Before using an alembic, be sure to check your local legislation that may not allow you to distil alcohol using an alembic.**

An alembic is a still to distil waters and oils from herbs. Pottery ones have been found by archaeology in Britain, but pewter or lead ones are recorded during the fourteenth century, although if the lead gets into the liquid, it is not going to be good for your long-term health. An alembic is a pot with an open bottom and a spout that points downwards out of the side. Inside the pot there is a section that runs around the base and part way to the top. The vapour rises from a container, into the alembic and condenses on the upper surface. It then runs down as a liquid to the internal rim and out of the spout into a container. These are often shown in pictures of an apothecary's garden. In fact, it is better to be indoors to have a good control of the environment. The alembic stands on top of a container with the liquid to be distilled. The plant parts should be crushed in a mortar and mixed with either water or white wine. The join between the lower pot and alembic should be completely sealed. A piece of wet linen cloth will usually do the job, but clay or bread dough is also good. The main difficulty is preventing the alembic from getting too hot, and it is usually necessary to keep it cool by regularly dabbing a wet cloth on it to allow the vapour to condense inside. This is important as it is an open system, and if care isn't taken, then the vapour may be lost. This was especially important when taking the alcohol off from wine, as the alcohol content of wines at this period was likely to be low compared to modern wines. The first few drops should not be collected as they are likely to be impure.

TO MAKE AQUA VITAE

Take white wine of Orsay and ginger, cloves, mace, kermes, cinnamon, a little pepper, galingale, a little sugar, cubebs (Piper cubeba), betony, tormentil, smallage, apium, mouse ear, scabious, bugle and violet. Grind the herbs small in a mortar. Bring them to the boil in a clean vessel with wine, then put them in a still, and distil them four or five times until the liquid will wet a linen cloth without staining it. Then take the liquid and put it in a glass.

If you are not legally allowed to use an alembic to distil spirits, you can add your plant material to a flavourless shop-bought spirit, such as vodka. Keep the vessel in

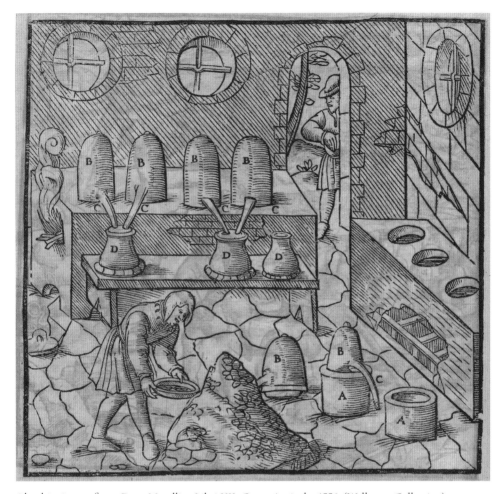

Alembics in use, from, De re Metallica Libri XII. Georg Agricola, 1556. (Wellcome Collection)

a cool and dark place. Shake once a day. In the earlier medieval period, the alcohol was wine, and the medicine would not keep for more than a few weeks. Once spirits were being distilled, tinctures could be kept for several years. If you did not have an alembic, you could use something more readily to hand.

TO MAKE ROSEWATER

Take a barber's basin and cover it with a cloth, like a drumhead. Lay the rose petals on the cloth. Above the rose have another basin of hot charcoal. Two glass basins can be used, but instead of burning charcoal, simply place the basins in the hot sun.

CHAPTER 14

Fun things to do

Make a Floral Chaplet

Floral chaplets, or crowns, are known to have been worn for festive occasions since at least the Roman period. They continued to be worn beyond medieval times and were worn by both women and men, lay people and by those of the church. There are many manuscript illustrations showing ladies collecting rose flowers from the garden and making coronets. It is difficult to see how the circlets were constructed, but the woman usually appears to be binding the flowerheads onto a frame made of thin twigs bent and tied into a circle, similar to the method used by modern florists. The flowers would have a short life span, but it probably didn't matter. Having experimented with different types of wood, the frame can be made using freshly cut willow withies or butcher's broom that has been left for a few days after cutting, otherwise it tends to be too brittle. Gently flexing the wood, bend the withy into an oval, then bind the ends with thread to the size you need. Overlap the ends by about five centimetres as this stops the ends from trying to move outwards. Make three hoops, place one on top of the other, making sure that the ends are staggered around the circle and do not line up, then using a threaded darning needle, bind the hoops together by weaving several times back and forth and tie a secure knot. Do this in about eight places to make a secure frame. Pick freshly opened roses on about 8 centimetres of stem. Remove any thorns. Starting at the front, tie along piece of thread to the frame, then place a rose flower on the outside of the frame and wrap the thread around the frame and stem. Repeat this until you run out of thread, tie off, then continue with a new thread. Medieval illustrations most commonly show alternate red and white flowers. The roses will last a few hours at most, but as the medieval poet wrote, 'Life is transient, like a mid-summer rose.' The frame can be reused with fresh roses. If you prefer, you can buy a modern wire frame instead. The red roses that I used for my crown were the red rose, *Rosa gallica*, the white rose is *Rosa alba semiplena* and the multi-coloured rose is Rosamundi.

Chaucer speaks of a garland made of marigolds in the Knight's Tale. Marigold stems are quite brittle, so the flowers could be tied to a frame or possibly a cord. An easy method relies on the flower stems to make a sturdy frame; take a flower stem, lay the next stem on top of the first, at ninety degrees to it.

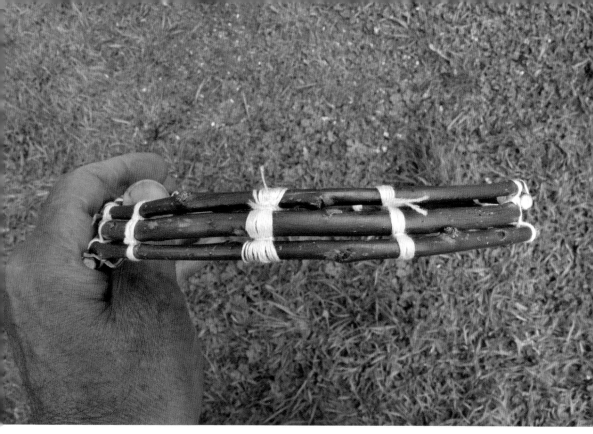

Above: A frame for a floral chaplet.

Below: Chaplet made of early historic roses.

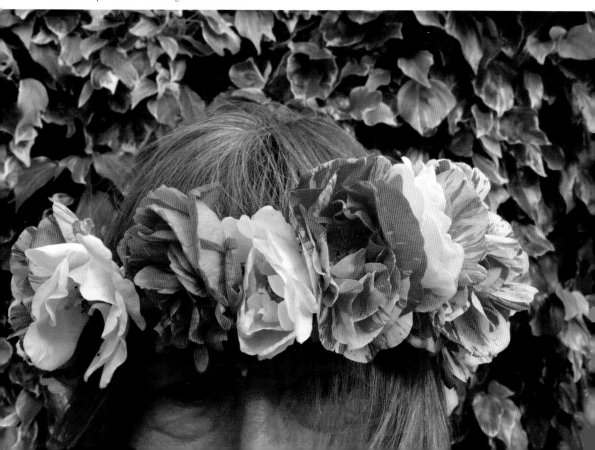

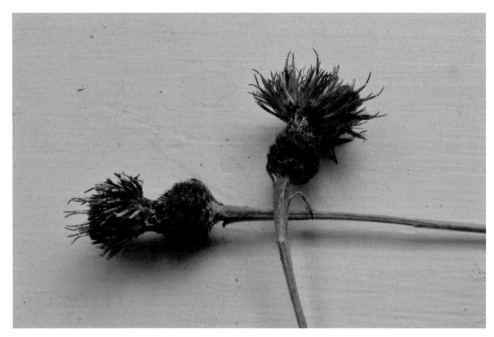

Floral Chaplet. Stage 1.

Space the flowerhead to suit the size of your flowers.

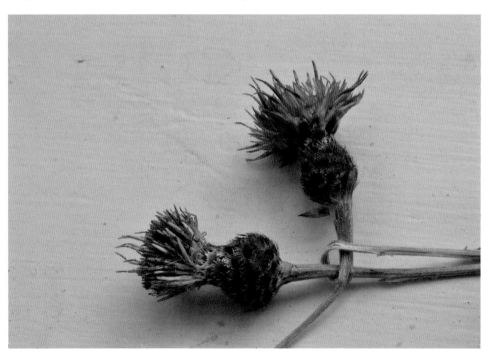

Floral Chaplet. Stage 2.

Wrap the stem of the second flower behind the first stem and behind its own flowerhead, pull the stem tight and lay it next to the first stem. Continue the process until the chain is long enough to fit your head, then tie the ends together with a spare plant stem, long grass or a piece cord. It is much easier to do it than to explain.

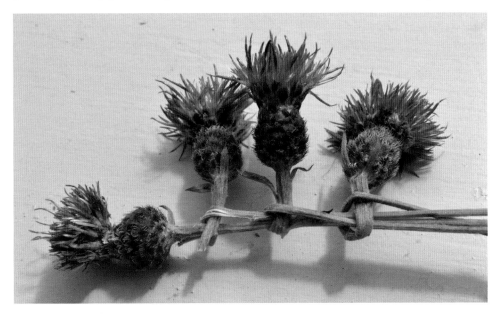

Above: Floral Chaplet. Stage 3.

Below: A completed chaplet using a selection of wildflowers.

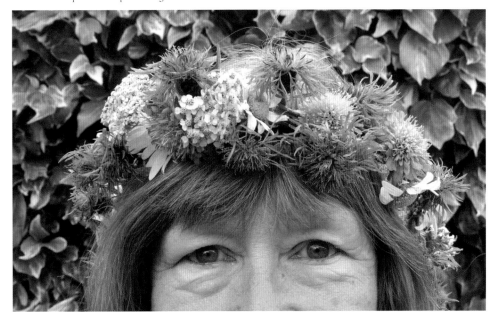

The simple daisy chain, where you make a slit below the flowerhead with a fingernail and push the next daisy stem through the hole, can be used for most herbaceous flowers; all you need is a sharp fingernail.

Musical instruments

Most musical instruments of the medieval period were made of wood, and took some time to construct, but some were very easy. In the late thirteenth century English song, *Ye have so longe keepyt the sheep*, the love says of the shepherd, Wilikin, her beloved, that he can make a good pipe with two rye straws. Pick a long stem of straw and cut it to make an open tube. You can cut finger holes if you wish. Cut another tube of straw two centimetres long and pinch one of the ends together, to make an oboe-like double reed and insert this into one end of the longer tube, and blow. You can make the instrument using only one stem by squashing the end together. Many modern wheat and barley stems are short, and narrow compared to the older and taller varieties, making this a fiddly and difficult instrument to make. It is much easier to cut a dried section of a teasel stem, just above a node so that one end is closed off, and then to shorten the tube to about fifteen centimetres. Place a sharp knife at right angles to the stem about a centimetre from the closed end. Carefully cut down until the knife has gone through the outer part of the stem, then cut horizontally for about four centimetres to make a thin tongue. Place the closed end of the stem in your mouth and close your lips to allow the air to escape only through the tube.

Ensure that the teasel tongue is free to vibrate. Blow gently. If there is no sound, vary the strength of blowing or wriggle the tongue to help it vibrate. If this does not work, scrape off a little of the tongue. It is sometimes easier to begin the cut four or so centimetres below the closed end and cut towards it as the tongue will not be able to split any further. Finger holes can be cut into the stem at an equal distance to produce a musical scale of sorts. It is a fun disposable instrument, but many ancient instruments use a similar reed. The drone reeds of bagpipes are made in a similar fashion.

In the medieval French song, *En Mai*, the poet has risen early to celebrate May Day:

In May, when the nightingale
sings cheerfully in the verdant bushes,
Then I must make a flageolet.
I shall make it of a willow twig,
As I must play on my flageolet concerning love,
And wear a chaplet of flowers.

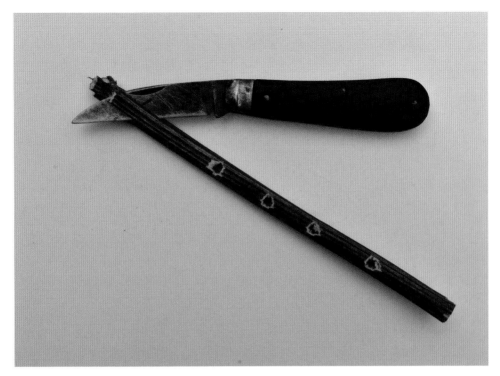

Cutting the tongue and a close-up of the tongue held open. It is usually more closed than this when about to play.

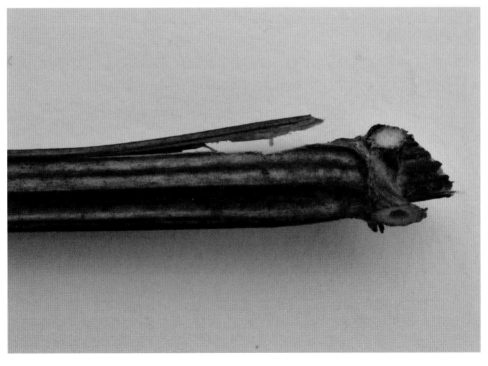

Willow whistles are best made when the sap is flowing fast in the spring. I made these as a child. Cut a length of willow with no side branches. A centimetre from the narrow end, cut down just into the wood, then move the blade about 3mm further down the stem and cut diagonally towards the first cut. Gently tap all the parts of the bark with a round piece of wood to loosen it; twist it carefully until it is fully loose, then gently pull the wooden core out from the wider end. Carefully slice a flat section from the mouthpiece end and cut downwards, completely through the wood from where you made the first vertical cut. Re-insert this short section, flat surface uppermost into the mouthpiece end. The end of this piece of wood should be in line with the vertical cut in the bark and not obstruct it. Blow through the mouthpiece to produce a note. If there is no sound close the bottom end with a finger; the mouthpiece block may need adjusting to get a strong note. The long piece can be put back in from the bottom and pulled in and out like a Swanee whistle, until the bark dries out. Finger holes can be made if you wish.

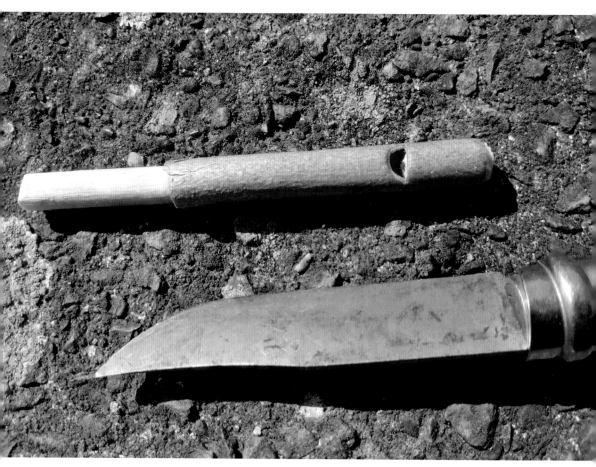

A willow whistle ready for playing.

CHAPTER 15

Plant Lists

Until Linnaeus perfected the scientific system of naming plants so that no matter where you are in the world, every plant had its own unique name, it was not always certain which plant was intended by the author. Most plants have common names that are identical to plants that are completely different. The descriptions of plants in some herbals are equally unhelpful. Most of the early herbals originated from ancient Mediterranean cultures. A western European scribe may have never seen or even heard of the plant that he is reading about, nor have any idea of what the plant looked like. This made the misidentification of a plant easy. The earlier drawings and later woodcuts were often inaccurate and may simply have shown a very generalised plant. Even if the original drawing had been accurate, as successive scribes copied the pictures the accuracy would tend to decrease. When artists, especially the later ones, drew from life, their drawings of plants or insects are easily identifiable. Scribal errors were easy to make, and understandable, so that even today, we are still not certain of the identity of some of the plants in medieval and earlier lists. Plants that today we consider to be quite different, were often thought to be the same or similar, *fleur-de-lys*, literally, the lily flower, usually refers to the iris, and the iris family of plants were treated as lilies for centuries to come.

I have given the modern botanical name to ensure the correct identity of the plant of the plant to which I am referring. The medieval names have been collated from several sources.

The following lists are the plants that are commonly mentioned in medieval herbals and literature. Not all were necessarily grown in British gardens and many attractive wild plants were probably collected from the countryside to be grown in the garden and not recorded as garden plants or being grown. Plants may be mentioned in the herbals, but there is no guarantee that they were grown in Britain, as some would not thrive because of the climate. Other plants that do not appear in formal writings can be found in ledgers of expenses and income that record seeds and plants being bought or sold, the maintenance costs of garden areas and the fruits of the harvest being sold. With some research we can have a good idea of the plants that were being grown during the medieval period. Some common plants of the countryside are not included because they were not mentioned at the time, for example, the red and white campions and field geraniums.

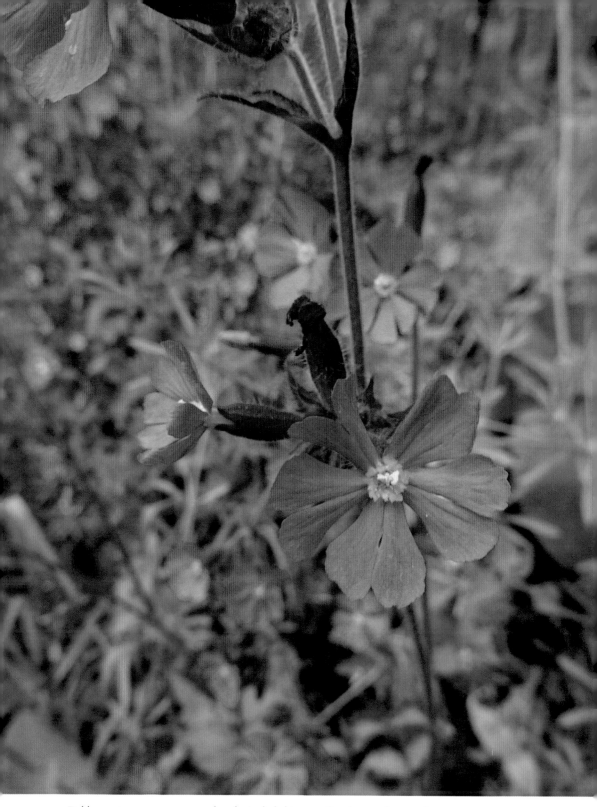

Field campions are pretty enough to be included in a medieval or modern garden.

  MEDIEVAL PLANTS AND THEIR USES

Rather than a long list, I have divided the plants into groups of their primary purpose, although many will have several uses. Whatever the medical or practical uses of the plants, most of them are very attractive, whether for their flowers, foliage, colour, scent or texture and many were grown in pleasure gardens for their beauty alone. Many of the plants can survive a reasonable amount of neglect. The plants that produce essential oils tend to be resistant to pests and generally the plants have the sort of flowers preferred by pollinating insects.

Most of the following plants are readily available as plants from nurseries or as seed and are quite easy to grow.

Herbs

Common Name	Botanical Name	Medieval Name	Uses
Agrimony	*Agrimona eupatoria*	Agrimonia. Egremoine. Egrimonye. Egrimoyne.	Medicinal.
Alecost. Costmary.	*Chrysanthemum balsamita*	Balsamita. Cost. Costus. Saint Mary.	Brewing. Medicinal.
Ammi	*Ammi majus*	Ameios. Amiens. Amiyis.	Medicinal.
Anise, Aniseed	*Pimpinella anisum*	Anise. Anisoum. Anneys. Anyse.	Culinary. Medicinal.
Avens	*Geum urbanum*	Auencia. Auence. Benedicta. Herb Benett.	Medicinal.
Baldmoney	*Meum athamanticum*	Spignel. Spigurnele.	Medicinal.
Balm, Lemon	*Melissa officinalis*	Bawme. Mellisa. Melisse.	Culinary. Medicinal.
Betony	*Stachys officinalis*	Betayn. Betonia. Betonica. Betonye. Betoyne. Boyshopyswort.	Medicinal.
Borage	*Borago officinalis*	Borage.	Culinary. Medicinal.
Bugle	*Ajuga reptans*	Bigula. Bugle.	Medicinal.
Bugloss	*Echium vulgare*	Bugle. (A common confusion).	Culinary. Medicinal.
Burnet	*Sanguisorba officinalis*	Burnete. Burnette.	Medicinal. Culinary.
Calamint	*Calamintha* spp.	Calamynt.	Medicinal.
Catmint	*Nepeta cataria*	Catys Mynte. Nepta. Nepte. Nepys.	Medicinal.

Common Name	Botanical Name	Medieval Name	Uses
Celandine, Greater	*Chelidonium majus*	Celidone. Celidonie. Celydonye. Teterwort.	Medicinal.
Centaury	*Erythroea centaureum*	Centaure. Centorie. Centory. Centorye	Medicinal.
Chamomile	*Anthemis nobilis*	Camamil. Camamilla. Camomil. Camomille. Camamylle.	Medicinal.
Cinquefoil	*Potentilla reptans*	Cincefoile. Fyfleued Grass. Quinque Folium.	Medicinal.
Clary Sage	*Salvia sclarea*	Sclarye. Clary.	Medicinal.
Clary, Field	*Salvia pratensis*	Sclarye.	
Coltsfoot	*Tussilago farfara*	Pes Pulli Agrestus. Folys Foot. Pes Pully.	Medicinal.
Comfrey	*Symphytum officinale*	Comfery. Consoude. Cumferie.	Medicinal.
Cornflower	*Centaurea cyanus*	Blew	Decorative.
Cowslip	*Primula veris*	Herbe of the Palsey.	Culinary. Decorative.
Daffodil	*Narcissus pseudonarcissus*	Affadilla. Affadille. Bell Blome.	Medicinal. Decorative.
Daisy	*Bellis perennis*	Dayesye. Petite Consoude. Ye of Day.	Culinary. Medicinal.
Dandelion	*Taraxacum officinalis*	Dendelyoun. Dens leonis. Lyons toth.	Culinary. Medicinal.
Dittander	*Lepidium latifolium*	Ditayne. Dytayne.	Medicinal.
Elecampane	*Inula helenium*	Elena. Elena Capana. Elene Campana. Elenium. Horsehelne. Horshillere.	Medicinal.
Eyebright	*Euphrasia officinalis*	Eufrace. Eufrasia. Eyebright.	Medicinal.
Fern, Common Polypody	*Polypodium vulgare*	Polipodi. Polipodie. Pollipodie.	Medicinal.
Fern, Female	*Athyrium filix-femina*	Feren.	Medicinal.

Common Name	Botanical Name	Medieval Name	Uses
Fern, Hart's Tongue	*Phyllitis scolopendrium*	Hartistonge. Hertestonge. Hertystungge. Lyngua cerui. Cerflange.	Medicinal.
Fern, Maidenhair	*Adiantum capillus-veneris*	Meiden-here.	Medicinal.
Fern, Male	*Dryopteris filix-mas*	Feren.	Medicinal.
Fern, Royal	*Osmunda regalis*	Osmund.	Medicinal.
Feverfew	*Chrysanthemum parthenium*	Febrefuga. Febri-fuga. Fetherfoy. Feverfew.	Medicinal.
Fleabane	*Pulicaria dysenterica*	Policaria. Policarie.	Medicinal. Strewing.
Forget-me-not	*Myosotis*	Me n'oubliez pas.	Symbolic.
Fumitory	*Fumaria officinalis*	Fumetere. Fumiter.	Medicinal.
Galingale	*Cyperus longus*	Ciperi.	Culinary.
Geranium, Dove's foot	*Geranium molle*	Pes Columbe	Medicinal.
Geranium, Herb Robert	*Geranium robertianum*	Herb Robert. Matwourth. Spragus.	Medicinal.
Germander	*Teucrium chamaedrys*	Camedreos. Gamandrea. Gamodreos. Germandria. Polium.	Medicinal.
Gromwell	*Lithospermum officinale*	Granium. Gromel. Gromelye. Lytyl Wale.	Medicinal.
Ground Ivy	*Glechoma hederacea*	Ale Hoof. Hayhove. Ere Terrestre.	Brewing. Medicinal.
Groundsel	*Senecio vulgaris*	Groundeswely. Groundswili. Growndswthele. Senacion.	Medicinal.
Heartsease	*Viola tricolor*	Pansy.	Decorative. Symbolic.
Hollyhock	*Althaea rosea*	Altea. Holy-Hok.	Medicinal. Decorative.
Holy Thistle	*Silybum marianum*	Thistil.	Medicinal.
Horehound, White	*Marrubium vulgare*	Horhoune. Horhowne. Horrowne. Houndbene. Marube. Marubium	Medicinal.

Common Name	Botanical Name	Medieval Name	Uses
Hounds Tongue	Cynoglossum officinale	Houndistonge. Houndistungge. Lingua canis.	Medicinal.
Houseleek	Sempervivum tectorum	Barbe Jovis. Hous leke. Semperviva. Sengrene. Sygrene.	Medicinal.
Hyssop	Hyssopus officinalis	Isopus. Ysop. Ysope.	Culinary. Medicinal.
Iris, German	Iris germanica	Flour-de-Lys. Flourdelys. Ireos. Irus.Yreos.	Medicinal.
Iris, Orris	Iris florentina	Ireos. Orris. Yreos.	Medicinal. Perfumery fixative.
Iris, Stinking	Iris foetidissima	Gladden. Gladene. Gladwyn. Ireos. Yreos.	Medicinal. Decorative.
Iris, Yellow	Iris pseudacorus	Flour-de-Lys. Flourdelys. Ireos. Irus. Yreos.	Medicinal.
Lady's Mantle	Alchemilla vulgaris	Pedelion. Lion's Foot.	Medicinal.
Lavender	Lavandula spica	Lavandula. Lavandre. Lavendre.	Cosmetic. Culinary. Medicinal.
Lavender, French	Lavandula stoechas	Sticados. Stickadove.	Culinary. Medicinal.
Lily, Madonna	Lilium candidum	Lilie. Lylium.	Medicinal. Symbolic.
Liquorice	Glycyrrhiza glabra	Licorys. Licoryce. Licoricia, Licoris, Lycoryse. Lyqueres. Liquoris.	Medicinal.
Loostrife, Yellow	Lysimachia vulgaris	Herbe Seint Christofere.	Medicinal.
Lovage	Levisticum officinale	Lovage.	Culinary. Medicinal.
Lungwort	Pulmonaria officinalis	Lungewort. Pulmonya. Pulmonye.	Medicinal.
Mallow	Malva sylvestris	Hockys. Malowe. Malva. Malve. Malwe. Okkys.	Medicinal.
Mallow, Marsh	Althaea officinalis	Altea. Bismalve. Holy-Hock.Holy-Hok. Wylde Malwe. Vyldemalwe.	Medicinal.
Marigold, Corn	Chrysanthemum segetum	Golds.	Decorative.

Common Name	Botanical Name	Medieval Name	Uses
Marigold, Pot	*Calendula officinalis*	Golds. Goldes. Marigoldys. Roddys. Rodewort. Solesqium.	Culinary. Medicinal.
Meadowsweet	*Filipendula ulmaria*	Filipendula. Reine.	Culinary. Medicinal. Strewing.
Meadow Clary	*Salvia pratense*	Oculus Christus. Oculus Christi.	Medicinal.
Mugwort	*Artemisia vulgaris*	Arthemesia. Moderwort. Mug-Wede. Mugwort. Mugwourth.	Brewing. Medicinal.
Mullein	*Verbascum thapsus*	Moleyn. Molayne. Moleyne. Soft.	Lighting. Medicinal.
Orchid	*Orchis mascula*	Saturion maior. Serapinum. Standelwhelkes. Yekes.	Medicinal.
Pellitory-on-the-Wall	*Parietaria diffusa*	Piretre. Peritorie.	Medicinal.
Pennyroyal	*Mentha pulegium*	Churche wort. Pulogium real. Puliole regale.	Culinary. Medicinal.
Peony, Female Peony, Male	*Paeonia officinalis* *Paeonia macula*	Piania. Pionre. Pyanye. Pyonye. Pyanye.	Medicinal.
Periwinkle	*Vinca minor*	Parvencis.	Medicinal. Chaplets.
Pink, Carthusian	*Dianthus carthusianorum*	Gelofre. Gillyflower.	Decorative.
Pink, Cheddar	*Dianthus gratianopolitanus*	Gelofre. Gillyflower.	Decorative.
Pink, Deptford	*Dianthus armeria*	Gelofre. Gillyflower.	Decorative.
Pink, Gillyflower	*Dianthus* spp.	Clowe Gelofre.	Culinary. Decorative. Medicinal.
Plantain, Greater	*Plantago major*	Plantayn. Planteyn the More. Waybrode.Weybread.	Medicinal.
Plantain, Lesser	*Plantago lanceola*	Launcele. Plantago minor. Plaanteyn the lasse. Rybwort.	Medicinal.
Poppy, Field	*Papaver rhoeas*	Wylde Poppy. Rede Popi.	Medicinal.
Primrose	*Primula vulgaris*	Plemeros. Primerole.	Decorative. Culinary.

Common Name	Botanical Name	Medieval Name	Uses
Rose, Dog	*Rosa canina*	Rose.	Decorative.
Rose, Red	*Rosa gallica var. officinalis*	Rosa Rubea. Rede Rose.	Cosmetic. Culinary. Decorative. Medicinal.
Rose, Sweet Briar	*Rosa eglanteria*	Rose. Egalantine.	Decorative. Culinary.
Rose, White	*Rosa alba*	Rose. White Rose.	Decorative. Medicinal.
Rosemary	*Rosmarinus officinalis*	Rosmarine. Rosmaryn.	Cosmetic. Culinary. Decorative. Medicinal.
Sage	*Salvia officinalis*	Salgia. Sauge. Salgea. Save. Saluia. Sawge	Culinary. Medicinal.
Sanicle	*Sanicula europaea*	Sanicle. Sanycle.	Medicinal.
Savory, Summer.	*Satureia hortense*	Saturea. Saueroye. Saverey. Saturia.	Culinary. Medicinal.
Scarlet Pimpernel	*Anagalis arvensis*	Chekenmete.	Medicinal.
Sedum.	*Sedum telephium*	Orpine. Orpyn. Orpyne. Fics-Herbe.	Medicinal.
Selfheal	*Prunella vulgaris*	Selfhele.	Medicinal.
Shepherd's Purse	*Capsella bursa-pastoris*	Bursa Pastoris. Sheppardis Purse.	Medicinal.
Solomon's Seal	*Polygonatum multiflorum*	Sigilium Sancte Marie. Seynt Marie Seal.	Medicinal.
Southernwood	*Artemisia abrotanum*	Abrotanum. Sothernwode. Sotherwode.	Medicinal. Strewing.
Spearwort	*Ranunculus lingua*	Lanceola. Sperewyrt.	Medicinal.
Stocks	*Matthiola incana*	Stock Gillyflower.	Decorative.
Strawberry	*Fragaria vesca*	Fragra. Streberye. Bleryd eyne. Streberywyse.	Culinary. Medicinal.
Sweet Cicely	*Myrrhis odorata*	Costus.	Culinary.
Sweet Rocket	*Hesperis matronalis*	Eruca Blanc.	Decorative.
Sweet Woodruff	*Galium odoratum*	Hastilogia. Woderowe. Wodroffe	Strewing.
Thyme, Bush	*Thymus vulgaris*	Tyme.	Culinary. Medicinal.
Thyme, Creeping	*Thymus serpyllum*	Hilwort. Piliole Monteyn. Tyme.	Culinary. Medicinal.

Common Name	Botanical Name	Medieval Name	Uses
Valerian	*Valeriana officinalis*	Cleoborum. Valerian. Cetwele.	Medicinal.
Vervain	*Verbena officinalis*	Verveyn. Verveyne.	Medicinal.
Violet, Sweet	*Viola odorata*	Violette.	Culinary. Medicinal.
Wallflower	*Cheiranthus cheiri*	Gillyflower.	Decorative.
Winter Savory	*Satureia montana*	Saturea. Saueroye. Saverey. Saturia.	Culinary. Medicinal.
Waterlily, White	*Nymphaea alba*	Nenufare.	Medicinal.
Waterlily, Yellow	*Nuphar, lutea*	Nenufare.	Medicinal.
Wood Anemone	*Oxalis acetosella*	Alleluia. Alleluya. Cuckoo's Bread. Gowk's Meat. Panis cuculi. Stoupwort. Stopwourt. Wodsour. Wodesowr. Woodsowr.	Medicinal.
Yarrow	*Achillea millefolium*	Millefolie. Milefoile. Mylefoyle.	Medicinal.

Culinary

Most of the culinary plants had medicinal uses too. Some of the leaves that were eaten are not considered to be palatable to modern tastes.

Common Name	Botanic Name	Medieval Name	Part Eaten
Alexanders	*Smyrnium olusatrum*	Alexandrum. Alysaundre. Stanmarch. Saunders.	Leaf. Root. Stem.
Basil	*Ocimum basilicum*	Basilicon. Ozmi.	Leaf.
Beets	*Beta vulgaris*	Betha. Betys. Beta. Bete.	Leaf. Root.
Broad Beans	*Vicia faba*	Beenez. Bene. Benez.	Seed.
Cabbage	*Brassica oleracea*	Caulus. Cool. Coleworts. Wortys. Worts. Wourte.	Leaf.
Caraway	*Carum carvi*	Carvi. Careway.	Culinary. Medicinal.
Carrot	*Daucus carota*	Dauke.	Root.
Celery, Wild	*Apium graveolens*	Apium. Smalach. Smalache. Merche.	Leaf.

Common Name	Botanic Name	Medieval Name	Part Eaten
Chervil	*Anthriscus cerefolium*	Apium risus. Cerfoylle. Chirfelle	Leaf.
Chicory	*Cichorium intybus*	Cicori.	Leaf.
Chives	*Allium schoenoprasum*	Chives.	Leaf. Flowers.
Cinnamon	*Cinnamomum verum or C. cassia*	Canel. Canell. Cynamomm.	Bark. Medicinal.
Coriander	*Coriandrum sativum*	Coliandrum. Colyandre. Coriandre. Coryandyr. Coriaundre.	Leaf. Seed. Medicinal.
Cress, Penny	*Lepidium sativum*	Cress.	Leaf.
Cumin	*Cuminum cymimum*	Comyn.	Seed.
Dill	*Anethum graveolens*	Anete. Anetum. Dille.	Leaf. Seed. Medicinal.
Fennel	*Foeniculum vulgare*	Fenel. Fenell. Feniculus. Fenkele.	Culinary. Medicinal.
Fenugreek	*Trigonella foenum-graecum*	Femygrek. Femygre. Fenigre. Fenigreke. Fenygrek.	Seed.
Garlic	*Allium sativum*	Alium. Garleek. Garlek. Cherlys Trycal. Cherlys Tryacle.	Bulb.
Gith	*Nigella sativa*	Git. Gith.	Seed.
Good King Henry	*Chenopodium bonus-henricus*	All Good. Mercurialis. Mercury. Mercurye.	Leaf. Seed.
Leek	*Allium porrum*	Porrum. Lek. Leke.	Bulb. Leaf.
Lettuce	*Lactuca sativa*	Lactuca. Letuse. Slepwourt.	Leaf.
Mint	*Menthe* spp.	Menta. Mynte.	Leaf.
Onions	*Allium cepa*	Cepe. Cep. Onyoun. Oynones.	Bulb.
Onions, Welsh	*Allium fistulosum*	Chibol. Ciboule.	Leaf.
Orache	*Atriplex hortensis*	Atriplex. Arage. Medles.	Leaf.
Oregano	*Origanum vulgare*	Organe. Origanum. Puliole Haunt.	Leaf.
Oxtongue, Bristly	*Picris echioides*	Langedbeef. Langdebef. Langedeboef. Lingua bovis. Longe de boef. Oxetunge. Oxtungge.	Leaf.

Common Name	Botanic Name	Medieval Name	Part Eaten
Parsley	*Petroselinum crispum*	Parsley. Parseli. Persil. Petrosilium.	Leaf.
Parsnip	*Pastinaca sativa*	Parsnepe.	Root.
Peas	*Pisum sativum*	Pees.	Seed.
Purslane	*Portulaca oleracea*	Porcelane. Purslayne. Portulake.	Leaf.
Radish	*Raphanus sativus*	Rappaner. Radich.Radiche.	Root.
Rocket	*Eruca sativa*	Eruca.	Leaf. Flowers.
Saffron	*Crocus sativus*	Safron. Safran.	Stamen.
Shallots	*Allium ascalonicum*	Onions of Ascalon.	Bulb.
Shepherd's Purse	*Capsella bursa-pastoris*	Bursa pastoris. Scheperdys purs. Schepehurdis poche. Tothwort.	Leaf.
Skirrets	*Sium sisarum*	Skyrwyt. Skyrwhit.	Root.
Sorrel	*Rumex acetosa*	Sorel. Sour-Doc.	Leaf.
Spinach	*Spinacia oleracea*	Spinage.	Leaf.
Watercress	*Rorippa nasturtium-aquaticum*	Watercresse. Watir Carses.	Leaf. Stem.
White Mustard	*Sinapis alba*	Rapistrum domesticum. Whitpepur.	Seed.

Tree and Bush Fruits

The list includes the most common trees that are found in medieval texts. Non-native fruit trees may have fruited well, but were commonly grown, e.g., peaches, except in warmer parts of Britain.

Common Name	Botanic Name	Medieval Name	Use
Almond	*Prunus amygdalus*	Alemandres. Almondis.	Culinary. Oil.
Apple, various	*Malus* spp.	Appil. Apple.	Cider. Culinary.
Bullace	*Prunus insititia*	Bolos.	Culinary.
Cherry	*Prunus avium*	Cheryse. Cheris.	Culinary.
Chestnut	*Castanea sativa*	Chesteyn.	Culinary. Timber.
Fig	*Ficus carica*	Fige. Fyg. Fygge.	Culinary. Medicinal.
Filbert	*Corylus maxima*	Filberdis.	Culinary.

Common Name	Botanic Name	Medieval Name	Use
Grapevine	*Vitis vinifera*	Vyne.	Wine.
Hazel Nut	*Corylus avellana*	Hasel. Hasil. Note.	Culinary.
Medlar	*Mespilus germanica*	Medler.	Culinary.
Mulberry	*Morus nigra*	Mores. Mylbery.	Culinary.
Pear	*Pyrus communis*	Pere. Peris.	Culinary. Perry.
Plum	*Prunus domestica*	Plumb. Ploume.	Culinary.
Quince	*Cydonia oblonga*	Citonie. Cowdris. Coynes.	Culinary.
Service Tree	*Sorbus domestica*	Aleys. Checkers.	Culinary.
Walnut	*Juglans regia*	Walis-Not. Walle-Notte. Walisshe-notis.	Culinary. Oil. Timber.

Trees and Shrubs

Common Name	Botanic Name	Medieval Name	Use
Alder	*Alnus glutinosa*		Pattens.
Ash	*Fraxinus excelsior*	Ash. Assh. Asshe.	Arrows. Pattens. Tool Handles.
Aspen	*Populus tremula*	Aspen.	Vine poles. Arrow shafts.
Bay	*Laurus nobilis*	Laure. Laurer. Lorer.	Culinary. Coronets. Medicinal.
Beech	*Fagus sylvatica*	Beche. Biche.	Timber.
Birch	*Betula* spp.	Birche.	Besom Brooms. Sap Wine.
Blackthorn	*Prunus spinosa*	Sloo. Blac Thorne.	Hedges.
Box	*Buxus sempervirens*	Boxtree.	Wind instruments.
Buckthorn	*Rhamnus catharticus*	Gaytree.	Medicinal.
Elderberry	*Sambucus nigra*	Elern.	Medicinal.
Elm	*Ulmus minor*	Elm. Elme.	Water Pipes.
Fir	*Picea abies*	Firre.	Ship's Masts.
Gorse	*Ulex europaeus*	Gorst.	Medicinal.
Hawthorn	*Crataegus monogyna*	Hawethorn. Thorne.	Hedges. Medicinal.

Common Name	Botanic Name	Medieval Name	Use
Holly	*Ilex aquifolium*	Holly.	Bird Lime.
Honeysuckle	*Lonicera periclymenum*	Caprifolium. Hony-sockles. Ligusticum. Wodebinde. Wodebynde. Wodbynd. Woodbyne. Wethwynde.	Medicinal.
Ivy	*Hedera helix*	Iuy.	Medicinal.
Juniper	*Juniperus communis*	Iuniper.	Culinary. Medicinal.
Lime	*Tilia cordata*	Linden. Lind.	Carved wood.
Maple	*Acer campestre*	Maple. Mapul.	Masers.
Myrtle	*Myrtus communis*	Mirte. Mirtille. Mirtus. Myrt.	Medicinal.
Oak	*Quercus robur*	Ook. Oke.	Buildings. Furniture.
Poplar	*Populus nigra*	Popler.	Timber.
Savin	*Juniperus sabina*	Savina. Savyn. Savyne. Saveyne.	Medicinal. Topiary.
Tutsan	*Hypericum androsaemum*	*Agnus Castus*. Tutsan. Parkleuys. Ypericon.	Medicinal.
Willow	*Salix* spp.	Saleyn. Salwe. Wilow.	Fencing. Baskets. Fish Traps. Bark and withies for tying. Medicinal.
Yew	*Taxus baccata*	Ew.	Bows.

Grains

Common Name	Botanic Name	Medieval Name	Use
Barley	*Hordeum vulgare*	Barly. Barlicche.	Culinary.
Oats	*Avena sativa*	Avena. Oates. Oatis.	Culinary.
Rye	*Secale cereale*	Rie.	Culinary.
Spelt	*Tricitum spelta*	Whete.	Culinary.
Wheat	*Tricitum aestivum*	Whete.	Culinary.
Wheat, Emmer	*Triticum dicoccum*	Whete.	Culinary.

Practical Plants

Common Name	Botanic Name	Medieval Name	Use
Butcher's Broom	*Ruscus aculeatus*	Ruge. (possibly!)	Brushes. Medicinal
Broom	*Cytisus scoparius*	Broum. Genescula.	Brooms. Medicinal.
Dyer's Greenweed	*Genista tinctoria*	Broum.	Yellow Dye
Flax	*Linum usitatissimum*	Flax. Flex. Lyne. Lynne. Lynseed,	Fibre. Linseed Oil.
Fullers Teasel	*Dipsacus sativus.* syn. D. *Fullonum* spp. *sativus*	Sheperdis Yeerd. Virga Pastoris.	Fulling woollen cloth.
Gourds	*Lagenaria vulgaris*	Gorde. Gourde.	Bottles. Containers. Medicinal.
Hemp	*Cannabis sativa*	Hempe.	Fibre. Medicinal.
Madder	*Rubia tinctorum*	Madir.	Red Dye. Medicinal.
Rush	*Juncus effusus*	Papyrus, called Paper.	Strewing. Lighting.
Soapwort	*Saponaria officinalis*	Saponaria. Crowsoth (Crows Soap). Soapwort. Fullers Herb.	Cleansing Cloth. Medicinal.
Weld	*Reseda luteola*	Weld.	Yellow Dye.
Woad	*Isatis tinctoria*	Gwayde.	Blue Dye. Medicinal.

Poisonous and Toxic Plants

Common Name	Botanic Name	Medieval Name	Use
Asarum	*Asarum europaeum*	Asarabaca Assarabacca. Azara.	Medicinal.
Belladonna	*Atropa belladonna*	Duscle. Dwale. More Morel. Solatrum nigrum.	Medicinal.
Birthwort	*Aristolochia rotunda*	Astrologie	Medicinal.
Caper Spurge	*Euphorbia lathyris*	Catapuce. Anabulla. Sporge	Medicinal.
Columbine	*Aquilegia vulgaris*	Cokkysfot. Columbina. Columbyne. Colverwort. Colverfot. Dowvesfot.	Medicinal.

Common Name	Botanic Name	Medieval Name	Use
Corncockle	*Agrostemma githago*	Gith. Cockle.	Medicinal.
Cuckoo Pint Lords and Ladies	*Arum maculatum*	Aaron. Cokkowyl pyntyl. Gotrampse. Iarus. Panis Cuculi.	Medicinal.
Dragons	*Dracunculus vulgaris*	Addyrwort. Dragaces. Dragansia. Dragauns. Dragancia femina. Dragans femel. Neddretunge. Oderwourt. Serpentyn.	Medicinal.
Foxglove	*Digitalis purpurea*	Glovewort.	Medicinal.
Hellebore, Black	*Helleborus niger*	Clowetungge. Ellebor. Ellebore. Ellebourus niger. Pedelyon.	Medicinal.
Hellebore, Stinking	*Helleborus foetidus*	Ellebore. Pedelyon.	Medicinal.
Hemlock	*Conium maculatum*	Cicuta. Hemloc. Hemelok.	Medicinal.
Henbane	*Hyoscyamus niger*	Henbane. Hennebane. Iusquiamus.	Medicinal.
Ivy	*Hedera helix*	Edere.	Medicinal.
Mandrake	*Mandragora officinarum*	Mandrage. Mandragore.	Medicinal.
Monkshood	*Aconitum nappellus*		Medicinal.
Mistletoe	*Viscum album*	Osinum. Mistilto.	Osinum. Mistilto.
Poppy, Opium	*Papaver somniferum*	Opie. Papauard.	Medicinal.
Rue	*Ruta graveolens*	Rawe. Rew. Rewe. Ruta domestica. Ruwe. Rw. Rwe. Ruw. Ryw. Rywe. Rue.	Medicinal.
Spurge Laurel	*Daphne laureola*	Lauriol. Lauriola. Laureole. Lauryol.	Medicinal.
Squill	*Urginea maritima*	Squylle. Scilla-de-morts-aux-rats.	Medicinal. Vermin.
St John's Wort	*Hypericum perforatum*	Herba Iohannis. Herbe Jon.	Medicinal.
Stavesacre	*Delphinium staphisagria*	Staphi. Stavesacre. Staves Acre. Lousewort.	Medicinal.

Common Name	Botanic Name	Medieval Name	Use
Tansy	*Tanacetum vulgare*	Tanesey. Tansey.	Strewing.
Dwarf Elder	*Sambucus ebulus*	Walwort.	Medicinal.
Wormwood	*Artemisia absinthium*	Warmode. Wormwood.	Medicinal. Strewing.
White Bryony	*Bryonia dioica*	Brionie. Briony. Nepe.	Medicinal.

For more information about medieval gardens and how they were maintained you may be interested in my previous book, *A Guide to Medieval Gardens. Gardens in the Age of Chivalry*, published by White Owl Books.

Further Reading

Albertus Magnus, Best, Michael R. and Brightman, Frank H., Eds., *The Book of Secrets of Albertus Magnus. Of the Virtues of Herbs, Stones and Certain Beasts, also a Book of the Marvels of the World.* Oxford University Press, 2004.

Arderne John, Power, D'Arcy, ed., *Treatises of Fistula in Ano*, Early English Text Society, 1968.

Bayard, Tania, *Sweet Herbs and Sundry Flowers, Medieval Gardens and the Gardens of the Cloisters*, The Metropolitan Museum of Art, Kingsworth Press, Tennessee, 1985.

Brodin, Gösta, *Agnus Castus. A Medieval English Herbal*, Harvard University Press, 1950.

Cato, *De Agricultura*, Dalby, Andrew, trans., Prospect Books, 1998.

Dawson, Warren, *A Leech Book*, or *Collection of Medical Recipes of the Fifteenth Century*, MacMillan and Co., Ltd, 1934.

Dioscorides, Gunther, Robert T, ed., *The Greek Herbal of Dioscorides*, Hafner Publishing company, London and New York, 1968.

Edmonds, John, *The History of Woad and the Medieval Woad Vat*, John Edmonds Publisher, 2000.

Frisk, Gösta, ed., *A Middle English Translation of Macer Floridus Herbarium*, Uppsala, 1945.

Gilbertus Anglicus, Getz, Faye Marie, ed., Healing and Medicine in Medieval England. A Middle English Translation of the Pharmaceutical Writings of Gilbertus Anglicus. The University of Wisconsin Press, 1991.

Green, Monica H, translated and edited, *The Trotula. An English Translation of the Medieval Compendium of Women's Medicine.* University of Pennsylvania Press, Philadelphia, 2002.

Hildegard von Bingen, Hozeski, Bruce W, trans., *Hildegard's Healing Plants*, Beacon Press Boston, 2001.

Hunt, Tony, *Popular Medicine in Thirteenth Century England*, D. S. Brewer Cambridge, 1994.

Keyte, Hugh, Parrott, Andrew, eds., *The New Oxford Book of Carols*, Oxford University Press, Oxford, 1992, reprinted 1994.

Pearsall, Derek, ed., *The Floure and the Leafe, The Assembly of Ladies, The Isle of Ladies*, Kalamazoo, Michigan: Western Michigan University for TEAMS, (Consortium for the Teaching of the Middle Ages, Inc.), 1990, second printing, 1992.

Pollington, Stephen, *Leechcraft. Early English Charms, Plantlore and Healing*, Anglo-Saxon Books, 2000.

Power, Eileen, *The Goodman of Paris (Le Menagier de Paris) A Treatise on Moral and Domestic Economy by a Citizen of Paris c. 1393*, The Folio Society, 1992.

Pughe, John, Trans., Williams Ab Ithel, Rev John, ed., *The Physicians of Myddfai*, Llanerch Publishers, 1993.

Ratti, Oscar and Westbrook, Adele, (translators), *The Medieval Health Handbook Tacuinum Sanitas*, George Braziller, New York, 1996.

Rawcliffe, Carole, *Medicine and Society in Medieval England*, Sandpiper Books, Sutton Publishing Ltd, 1995.

Stannard, Jerry, Stannard, Katherine E. and Kay, Richard eds., *Herbs and Herbalism in the Middle Ages and Renaissance*, Ashgate Publishing Limited, 1999.

Strabo, Walahfrid, *Hortulus*, Payne, Raef, trans., The Hunt Botanical library, Pennsylvania 1966.

van Arsdall, Anne, *Medieval Herbal Remedies. The Old English Herbarium and Anglo-Saxon Medicine*, Routledge New York and London, 2002.

Internet Sources

The Wellcome Collection. Digitised herbals and much else. https://wellcomecollection.org/

A Litil Bok of the Pestilence:
https://archive.org/details/litilbokewhichetoojoanrich/page/19/mode/1up

The Master of Game. Information on medieval hunting.
https://archive.org/details/masterofgameoldexxooedwa

All photographs were taken by the author unless otherwise stated. Special thanks to Patricia Hall for the photo of the carving of silphium, page 109.
The quote from the disgruntled monk complaining about eating peas every day is repeated from, *In a Monastery Garden*, by Elizabeth and Reginald Peplow. The verse is often quoted in other places, but so far, I have been unable to find the original source.

I would like to thank Janet Hays and Margaret Jones for their support, advice and help with the writing and editing of this book.
Special thanks to Sean Jones of Jones Instruments, Leek, Staffordshire for the idea of using teasel stems to make a simple musical instrument.